Writing Scientific Research in Communication Sciences and Disorders

Writing Scientific Research in Communication Sciences and Disorders

Robert H. Brookshire, PhD, CCC-SLP, F-ASHA
Shelley B. Brundage, PhD, CCC-SLP, BCS-F, F-ASHA

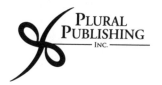
PLURAL
PUBLISHING
INC.

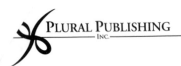

PLURAL PUBLISHING
INC.

5521 Ruffin Road
San Diego, CA 92123

e-mail: info@pluralpublishing.com
Website: http://www.pluralpublishing.com

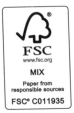

FSC
www.fsc.org
MIX
Paper from
responsible sources
FSC® C011935

Typeset in 10½/13 Palatino by Flanagan's Publishing Services, Inc.
Printed in the United States of America by McNaughton & Gunn, Inc.

For permission to use material from this text, contact us by
Telephone: (866) 758-7251
Fax: (888) 758-7255
e-mail: permissions@pluralpublishing.com

Library of Congress Cataloging-in-Publication Data

Brookshire, Robert H., author.
  Writing scientific research in communication sciences and disorders / Robert H.
Brookshire, Shelley B. Brundage.
     p. ; cm.
  Includes bibliographical references and index.
  ISBN 978-1-59756-614-8 (alk. paper)—ISBN 1-59756-614-4 (alk. paper)
  I. Brundage, Shelley B., author. II. Title.
  [DNLM: 1. Medical Writing. 2. Publishing. 3. Speech-Language Pathology.
WZ 345]
  R119
   808.06'661—dc23
                              2015022421

Contents

Foreword

This book is not about theory, not about a specific communication disorder, not about experimental design, and not about statistical analysis. It is about scientific writing—that part of research that tells a story about a problem that has been studied systematically, a story often driven by theory and organized around hypotheses, and structured by solid study design and methods of data collection and analysis. It is essentially the final act of any research endeavor, but typically the only act seen by students, clinicians, and researchers who hope to benefit from its publication.

Writing about research, or scientific writing, is no easy task and, in fact, has itself been a topic of considerable discussion in the scientific literature. It is well accepted—though not always evident in published research—that "the fundamental purpose of scientific discourse is not the mere presentation of information and thought, but rather its actual communication," and that just because science is often complex, it "need not lead to impenetrability of expression" (Gopen & Swan, 1990, p. 550).

Although there can be no fixed formula for good scientific writing, "in real and important ways, the structure of the prose becomes the structure of the scientific argument" (Gopen & Swan, 1990, p. 558). This reflects the close bond between clear thinking and clear writing and suggests that improving one may improve the other. At the same time, however, scientific writing is a special skill that does not automatically flow from clarity of thought; for most people, it requires focused attention and hard work to hone writing skills. If these statements seem too esoteric or vague, it may help simply to remember that editors and publishers are not in business to rewrite poorly written papers and that poorly written papers often raise concerns about clarity of thought and scientific merit. Authors who write clearly and efficiently have a leg up in the competition for space in journals.

In this book, Bob Brookshire and Shelley Brundage provide invaluable guidance for writing about research in communication sciences and disorders. They systematically address the content, structure, and style associated with each section of a scientific paper and the variety of approaches that can be used to write them well. You will find many concrete examples from published studies that illustrate how each section of a manuscript can convey the research story concisely and informatively. The chapters dealing with the construction of data tables and graphs not only will help decisions about how best to summarize data, they will also help you, the writer, identify and interpret the data that most directly address the questions posed in the study. Careful attention to the advice provided about the construction of the abstract and the title is strongly recommended, because they are what readers use to decide if allotting time to read beyond them might be of value; limited in length, you would think the title and abstract should be easy to construct, but speaking from my own writing struggles, they are not. Students will also want to pay close attention to the chapter on literature reviews, because it is broadly applicable to many academic papers you may be required to write, even if they do not involve experimental research. And, in my opinion, students and many experienced researchers will benefit from reading and then revisiting (perhaps repeatedly) the advice given in the chapters on content and copy editing. Failures at this stage of the writing process are often the source of manuscript rejection or harsh reviews, even in the presence of an important and well-designed and executed study or review paper.

Finally, before reading the book in a linear way, consider first reading the final two chapters (13 and 14) that address the peer review process and the writing process. They will give you a sense of the challenges—and strategies for meeting them—that are part of the journey that will put you in a position to share what you have learned with your professional colleagues.

For undergraduate and graduate students, *Writing Scientific Research in Communication Sciences and Disorders* should be a valuable resource whether or not you eventually embark on a career that will require you to write and publish the results of research. Clear writing is equally important in clinical and educational settings in which you must convey your observations, diagnoses, and recommendations for patients, clients, caregivers, students, and colleagues in written form. And, for those who are already working as researchers, clinicians, and teachers, I can attest from personal experience to the career-long need to refine writing skills; they are nearly inseparable from the continuing need to refine clinical and research skills. This book will serve as an aid to you, and to me, in that process.

—Joseph R. Duffy, PhD, BC-ANCDS
Emeritus Professor
Mayo College of Medicine
Member, Division and Section of
    Speech Pathology
Department of Neurology
Mayo Clinic
Rochester, Minnesota

Reference

Gopen, G. D., & Swan, J. A. (1990). The science of scientific writing. *American Scientist, 78*, 550–558.

Preface

It began innocently enough, with a memory of a writing seminar taught at the University of Minnesota, and the quest to convert the concepts and notes taught there into a book on writing. Dr. Robert Brookshire created that seminar, and this book is my attempt to capture the wisdom of that course and the book that he began.

Developing my own writing seminar at George Washington University took me back to Bob's course and to writing my doctoral dissertation under his expert guidance. I knew that he had been refining his course notes with a goal of publishing a book on writing, but he died before finishing it. Before he died, Bob asked that Joe Duffy review the manuscript and consider what could be done to shepherd the book into print. Joe and I discussed this and shared the files Bob had drafted. With them in hand, I eagerly agreed to take on the task of finishing the book.

Bob's files contained the core of this book, but they were not yet in a condition that he would have considered ready for publication. Some key chapters needed to be written, and existing chapters needed editing. Throughout the process I have asked myself repeatedly, "how would Bob write or rewrite this?" Finishing the book was a great way to get reacquainted with him. Perhaps that is a sign of excellent mentors: their guidance and ways of thinking remain with you long after the initial mentorship experience. Bob was one of those truly great teachers and mentors.

Bob Brookshire was a prolific and highly respected scholar in aphasiology, known for his skills in measuring complex human communication behaviors.

He authored over 50 peer-reviewed papers and mentored 22 master's thesis students and 12 doctoral students. He and his wife and collaborator, Linda Nicholas, published seminal articles on the auditory comprehension and verbal production abilities of persons with aphasia. Their work produced the Discourse Comprehension Test (Brookshire & Nicholas, 1993), a test to evaluate discourse comprehension in aphasia. Nicholas and Brookshire's correct information unit analyses continue to be used to quantify the speech production of persons with communication disorders. Bob was also the author of the widely adopted textbook, *Introduction to Neurogenic Communication Disorders*, now in its eighth edition.

Bob's commitment to clear scientific writing and his editorial skills were well known by students and colleagues. With his green pencil in hand (because "red looks too much like blood"), he would respond to many a students' thesis or dissertation with entreaties to find a "better word" or to "be clear and direct," often with the gentle comment, "I wonder how much of this you really need." As he reminded us often, findings that are not well communicated are essentially lost on the reader.

Bob received many awards during his long career, but of all the recognition he received, it was the Golden Shovel Award that held pride of place in his office. This award recognized his 20+ years as editor of the *Clinical Aphasiology Conference (CAC) Proceedings*, where his green pencil did the shoveling that made those proceedings clear and concise. Bob also served as an associate editor for two ASHA journals, the *Journal of Speech, Language, and Hearing Research* and the *Journal of Speech and Hearing Disorders*.

The goal of this book is not to teach you how to write. Chances are you already know how to do that. The purpose is to help you to write better, *and to do so for* *scholarly scientific publication*. I hope this book helps you to become a better writer, and to find your own writing voice. And I hope, as would Bob Brookshire, that by so doing, your contributions to scientific discourse will be clearly and concisely communicated.

—Shelley B. Brundage
Washington, DC

References

Brookshire, R. H., & Nicholas, L. E. (1993). *Discourse Comprehension Test*. Tucson, AZ: Communication Skill Builders.

Brookshire, R. H., & McNeil, M. R. (2015). *Introduction to neurogenic communication disorders*. St. Louis, MO: Elsevier Mosby.

Acknowledgments

I'll be honest, until I worked on this book, I never read the acknowledgments section. Now I read them all the time. I have a lot of people to thank, but I promise I will not go on and on like I won an Oscar or something.

First, I am very grateful to Linda Nicholas, for her support and her trust in me to bring this book to publication. Linda, thank you for believing I could do this, and for allowing me to honor Bob's work by doing so.

My husband Rich was steadfast in his support and willingness to help with any detail, none too big or small. Thank you especially for creating the index, wrestling with MSWord and WordPerfect, your editing skills, and for your willingness to eat pizza much more frequently than usual.

Joe Duffy served as an early advisor and mentor in the publishing process. Thank you, Joe, for helping me find Plural and for your advice on how to put a book proposal together. Thank you also for your assurances that you thought I could do this. That means a lot to me.

My department colleague Adrienne Hancock, herself an excellent and prolific scholar, kept me focused and talked me out of "writing rabbit holes" at some critical times during the last year. I continue to enjoy our conversations about teaching and writing.

I am grateful to my colleagues in the George Washington University Writing Program for our discussions about all aspects of teaching writing. Thank you to Randi Kristensen, Derek Malone-France, Rachel Riedner, and Phil Troutman.

The encouragement that I received from my writing group at Academic Ladder was invaluable and kept me focused on getting the book *done*. Thanks to all of you in Social Science Professors Group 5.

Everyone at Plural Publishing has been supportive and helpful. From my initial meeting with Valerie Johns, to Kalie Koscielak's informative e-mails and organized processes, it has been an educational and enjoyable experience for me.

Finally, thank you to my daughter Janetta, who thought it was "cool" that her mom was writing a book on writing, and even "cooler" that I was doing it to honor one of my teachers. Janetta, I think you are pretty cool, too. Let's not have pizza for dinner.

To Linda and to Rich, instrumental partners with Bob and me every step of the way.

1

Writing and Learning Are Complementary Activities

" . . . the act of writing . . . had clarified my half-formed ideas.
Writing and thinking and learning were the same process."

—Zinsser, 1988, ix

Students often ask me, "Why do I have to write a research paper for your class? When I am a working speech pathology professional, I will never have to write a paper like this!" My answer is that accurate, clear, and concise written communication is required for our professions. In addition, writing is a window on the depth of your understanding of a topic. In his book, *On Writing*, Steven King suggests that "writing is refined thinking" (King, 2000, p. 131), and I could not agree more. Writing helps you organize your thoughts.

Writing involves both internal and external conversations. Writers have internal, meta-cognitive conversations with themselves, asking "what do I know?" and "how do I know it?" This internal conversation helps writers to build their knowledge about a topic and see connections between topics. The conversation also allows writers to see where there are gaps in their knowledge, by asking questions such as "where does this topic fit in?" or "do I have evidence to back up that statement?" The act of writing allows you to apply your knowledge, integrate it with other topics, and reflect on what it means (Dunn, Saville, Baker, & Marek, 2013).

Writing is also an external conversation between the writer and the audience. Good writers know who their audience is, and they keep their audience's knowledge of the topic in mind as they write. For example, you would probably write differently if your audience was other speech-language pathologists (SLPs) than if your audience was parents of children with communication disorders. Most audiences prefer simple and direct writing, but what is simple changes with the audience.

The intended audience for this book is undergraduate and graduate students in Communication Sciences and Disorders (CSD). The information in this book may also be useful to other scholars or beginning researchers who are interested in making their writing more concise and clear.

What the Research Says About Writing and Learning

John Dewey (1916) wrote that students learn best when they are presented with real problems that they must solve, because these types of problems promote active learning and critical thinking. Writing formalizes this problem-solving and critical-thinking process, and in some ways writing is the framework in which we organize our thinking to solve the problem at hand. John Bean suggests that writing is a "product that communicates the results of critical thinking" (Bean, 2011, p. 4).

Across a variety of professional disciplines, writing assists adults in learning new information. Writing enhances learning in allied health fields such as nursing (Luthy, Peterson, Lassetter, & Callister, 2009; Schmidt, 2004), occupational therapy (Griffiths, Coppard, & Lohman, 2009), physical therapy (Williams & Wessel, 2004), and psychology (Radhakrishnan, Schmmack, & Lam, 2011). Writing allows you to formulate, state, and share your ideas with others.

The CSD professions require many types of writing. Clinical SLPs and audiologists write diagnostic reports, treatment plans, Individualized Education Plans, Individual Family Service Plans, insurance justifications—the variety of written output seems endless. Researchers and professors in CSD also write and review a variety of documents: curriculum-related documents, evaluations of student learning, lectures, examinations, and research papers.

Purpose of This Book

The purpose of this book is to describe how to write a research paper in CSD. The book contains chapters on each section of a research paper (Introduction, Method, Results, and Discussion). There are also chapters on aspects of the writing process, such as editing, creating figures and graphs, and peer review. We discuss different writing styles and provide examples of these styles. Although there are many different ways to write well, there are plenty of ways to write wrong! This book is meant to help you avoid some common pitfalls in professional writing.

The book begins with the Introduction chapter. This chapter explains the types of information that should be included in the Introduction section of a research paper, and describes different ways to present this information.

The chapter on the Method section provides guidance on how to describe your study's participants, materials used, and procedures. The Method section is where astute readers will go to evaluate the internal validity of your study. Readers will be looking for essential information on how your study was done; this chapter tells you what that information is and how to write about it.

Once your readers are convinced of the soundness of your methodology, they will want to know what you learned from it. The Results, Constructing Data Tables, and Constructing Data Graphs chapters explain how to present the findings of your study. The Results chapter also has a section on how to report some of the most commonly used statistics in CSD research.

The Discussion chapter explains how to write about the meaning and applicability of your results, and the generalizability of your findings. Here you will make the case for the significance of your study, and we explore some approaches and pitfalls in making your case.

The Title and Abstract chapters follow the Discussion, because these are best written last. It's much easier to write an abstract when you know the results and know what the results mean. The title and abstract of your paper are extremely important, as they form the first—and perhaps only—impression that the reader will have of your paper.

We then turn our attention to exploring specific aspects of the writing process. We first consider Literature Reviews, describing systematic reviews and meta-analyses, and seeing how these articles are different from standard research articles.

There are two chapters on editing. The first, Content Editing, explains how to look at your work from the perspective of an editor. This chapter describes ways to clarify the essential message of your work. The Copy Editing chapter is the distillation of over 60 years of experience in reading, writing, and editing research in CSD. Here you will find ideas, rules, and techniques to make your writing clear, concise, and persuasive.

The last two chapters are about getting your writing done and published. Getting Published describes the processes involved in getting your work published, including a discussion of peer review and how to work with editors. The Writing Process chapter has ideas and resources for getting started and keeping going. We also provide a list of resources that influenced our thinking about writing and teaching writing.

We include writing evaluation guidelines at the end of most chapters. Think of these guidelines as summaries of the chapter topics. Consider these self-evaluations prior to submitting your work for publication, or when you read the work of others.

References

Bean, J. (2011). *Engaging ideas: The professor's guide to integrating writing, critical thinking, and active learning in the classroom* (2nd ed). San Francisco, CA: Jossey-Bass.

Dewey, J. (1916). *Democracy and education: An introduction to the philosophy of education.* New York, NY: Free Press.

Dunn, D., Saville, B., Baker, S., & Marek, P. (2013). Evidence-based teaching: Tools and techniques that promote learning in the psychology classroom. *Australian Journal of Psychology, 65,* 5–13.

Griffiths, Y., Coppard, B., & Lohman, H. (2009). From pedestal to possibility: Learning scholarly writing using a unique course assignment. *Journal of Allied Health, 34,* 97–100.

King, S. (2000). *On writing.* New York, NY: Scribner.

Luthy, K., Peterson, N., Lassetter, J., & Callister, L. (2009). Successfully incorporating writing across the curriculum with advanced writing in nursing. *Journal of Nursing Education, 48,* 54–59.

Radhakrishnan, P., Schmmack, U., & Lam, D. (2011). Repeatedly answering questions that elicit inquiry-based thinking improves writing. *Journal of Instructional Psychology, 38,* 247–252.

Schmidt, L. (2004). Evaluating the writing-to-learn strategy with undergraduate nursing students. *Journal of Nursing Education, 43,* 466–473.

Williams, R., & Wessel, J. (2004). Reflective journal writing to obtain student feedback about their learning during the study of chronic musculoskeletal conditions. *Journal of Allied Health, 33,* 17–23.

Zinsser, W. (1988). *Writing to learn.* New York, NY: Harper & Row.

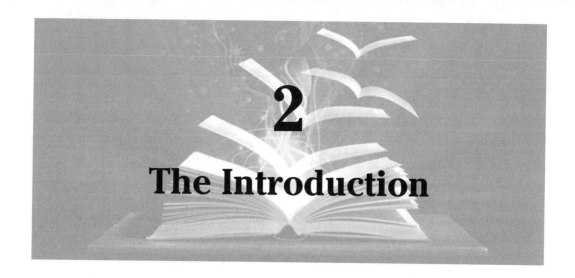

2

The Introduction

"The effective beginning . . . lets readers know what to expect but leaves them something to expect."

—Thomas Kane (1988)

The purpose of the introduction to a research report is to provide the background information readers need to appreciate the topic, purpose, and scope of the report. The introduction should include coverage of

- the problem area or research questions under study,
- the history of the problem area,
- the relationship of the research to existing knowledge,
- the purpose of the research described in the report, and
- the specific experimental questions addressed or hypotheses tested in the research.

Sternberg (1993) comments that the introduction to a research article should answer four basic questions:

- What previous research led to this research?
- What does this research add to previous research?
- Why is the addition made by this research important or interesting?
- How is the addition made?

Setting the Scene

Introductions to published research articles in the behavioral sciences, medicine, and related areas typically open with a general statement that places the research in a broad knowledge domain, as in the following examples:

- From a study of the effects of several variables on observers' judgments of the direction of eye gaze (Gamer & Hecht, 2007):

Knowing whether one is the recipient of a gaze—be it the gaze of a friend or of an enemy—can be decisive in many social interactions.

- From a study on bilingual listeners' recognition of English words in noise (Shi, 2015):

Speech perception is difficult to evaluate in bilingual listeners.

- From a study of relationships between performance on

neuropsychologic tests and driving performance of persons with Parkinson's disease (Stolwyk, Charlton, Triggs, Iansek, & Bradshaw, 2006):

The issue of driving competency in people with Parkinson's disease is controversial.

■ From a study of the effects of victim characteristics such as sex and occupation on jurors' judgments regarding the presence of mild traumatic brain injury (Guilmette, Temple, Kennedy, Weiler, Ruffolo & Dufresne, 2005):

Personal injury litigation for traumatic brain injuries has increased significantly in recent years.

Reviewing the Literature

From such general opening statements, introductions typically go on to provide a brief history of the problem area—a review of the relevant literature. The review places the current work in a domain of knowledge and helps readers appreciate the relationship of the current work to previous work. The review may summarize important previous work; describe important trends and common themes; identify misconceptions, contradictions, and inconsistencies in previous work; discuss unexplained relationships; or point out unresolved theoretical issues. The review takes readers from what is known about a problem area to what needs to be known (that is, what you intend to find out), and shows the logical relationships between previous work and the current work.

The review of literature may range from two or three paragraphs to three or four pages, depending on the complexity of the problem and the amount of attention given the problem in the past. Literature reviews typically follow a chronological pattern of development, beginning with early work in the problem area and progressing to the most recent work that relates to the question of interest. The chronology can be either single-topic or multiple-topic, depending on the complexity of the history of the question.

Most research articles focus on a specific question with a relatively narrow history; therefore, reviews of literature typically follow a single-topic chronological pattern of development in which the review progresses from the earliest significant works to the most recent. Headings usually are not needed in such single-topic reviews.

The history of research on some topics is more varied, representing different theoretical or philosophical directions, with different participants, measures, and methods. In such cases, a multiple-topic pattern of development is more appropriate. Topics representing clusters of works with a common theme are presented in separate chronological accounts. Headings often are needed to mark the topics in such multiple-topic reviews.

Here is an outline of a multiple-topic introduction to an article (Moberg & Curtin, 2009) describing an experiment that evaluated the effects of alcohol on fear and anxiety in human participants, in which the authors divide the introduction into four sections with the following headings:

■ *Alcohol use and stress,*
■ *Fear versus anxiety: Methods, mechanisms, and measures,*

■ *Alcohol and other drug effects on fear versus anxiety,* and
■ *The current study.*

In this example, the authors first summarize literature related to normal and problem drinkers' use of alcohol to reduce stress. Next, they describe how fear and anxiety have been differentiated in laboratory settings. They then summarize previous findings related to differential effects of alcohol and drugs on fear and anxiety. Finally, they tell how they plan to experimentally separate and measure the effects of alcohol on fear from its effects on anxiety, and they offer several hypotheses about what they expect to find. The introduction spans about two and a half journal pages.

The review of literature is not an annotated list of what has been written on the topic, arranged in chronological order. In addition to telling readers the history of the problem, the review of literature develops a logical framework that supports the rationale for the current study by showing how cited works relate to each other and to the present work.

Stating the Purpose

The introductions to most research articles close with statements of purpose. Here is the closing statement from Gamer and Hecht's (2007, p. 706) eye gaze study:

The experiments reported here were designed to examine two characteristics of this gaze cone, namely its width and its central direction, as a function of several variables. In contrast to the vast majority of studies cited above, we opted for an interactive quantitative

measure of the point where a given gaze is perceived to fall just inside the range that would be classified as looking at the observer.

Sometimes authors follow statements of purpose with hypotheses or predictions of expected results. Martin and McDonald (2005, p. 715) give the statement of purpose from a study of traumatically brain-injured persons' comprehension of ironic jokes, followed by the authors' hypotheses:

(Statement of Purpose) This study aimed to distinguish between two broad theoretical perspectives; first, that ToM [theory of mind] deficits account for irony comprehension deficits; i.e., a domain-specific account, and second, that both mentalizing deficits and poor irony comprehension are a result of a broader impairment to inferential reasoning, reflecting executive dysfunction secondary to frontal-lobe damage.

(Hypotheses) First, for a ToM account of pragmatic impairment in TBI to be supported, it was expected that the ability to reason about mental states (ToM) would be significantly associated with the ability to distinguish between ironic jokes and lies . . . Furthermore, given that ToM is argued to be a domain-specific account of pragmatic deficits, inference making more generally (i.e., non-mental inferences) would not predict the ability to comprehend irony.

Second, for an EF (executive function) account of irony comprehension to be supported, it was expected that ToM deficits would exist concurrently to general deficits in inferential reasoning. In addition, the ability to understand ironic jokes would be associated with (i) conceptual reasoning and flexibility and (ii) working memory.

In another example, the authors (Martinussen & Tannock, 2006, p. 1075) give the statement of purpose from a study of working memory impairments in children with attention-deficit hyperactivity disorders, followed by a summary of the results expected by the authors:

(Statement of Purpose) The primary aim of the present study was to evaluate verbal and spatial storage and C.E. [central executive] components of working memory in a sample of children with confirmed ADHD [attention-deficit hyperactivity disorder] while controlling for both comorbid reading difficulty (RD) and language impairment (LI) to better delineate the cognitive deficits specifically associated with ADHD. A second aim was to examine the association between working memory and the two behavioral dimensions of ADHD (inattention, hyperactivity-impulsivity).

(Expected Results) On the basis of this research we predicted that children classified as ADHD [attention-deficit hyperactivity disorder] Combined Type or Primarily Inattentive would exhibit similar working memory profiles and that both subgroups would be impaired relative to normal controls on the C.E. [central executive] components of working memory. Similarly, it was hypothesized that weaknesses in C.E. working memory functioning would be associated with symptoms of inattention but not with symptoms of hyperactivity-impulsivity.

Summary: How to Write the Introduction

The Opening: Setting the Stage

Readers will be asking, "what's the point," from the first words they read, so make your point obvious in the first few paragraphs. Identify the research problem you have chosen to investigate. Tell why the problem is important. Tell how your research adds to knowledge about the problem.

Writing the introduction is no time to be coy. You are not writing drama or a novel, so don't keep readers in the dark about where you are headed. Plan to establish the direction of your research in the first two or three paragraphs. Define any terms that may be unfamiliar to readers, and explain general concepts that may underlie your work. Provide enough background material to show the major connections between your work and previous work, but save detailed discussion of previous work and how your work relates to it for later in the introduction. When you have identified the problem under investigation and have provided enough explanatory material to ensure that readers understand what you are up to, you are ready to move on to more elaborate description of the literary and theoretical background of your work.

The Middle: Giving the Background

Here, as in other parts of the paper, readers appreciate brevity. Structure the content of the review of literature around your sense of what your readers are likely already to know about the topic. Most readers will have at least general knowledge of the literature relating to your work. They will not be interested in wading through tangential or irrelevant material to get your point. Discuss only enough background material to set the scene for the current work. Tie the background information to the purpose of the paper, and make the ties clear.

Include only works that are germane to your work. Do not take readers back to the beginnings of thought on the topic of your paper. Do not include work of general relevance or work that is tangential to your work. When you include previous work, discuss only those aspects of the work that you address in your paper —previous findings that relate directly to your theories and hypotheses; methodological issues that you intend to resolve; and conclusions that you intend to evaluate. Don't use the introduction to impress readers with the amount of time you spent researching the topic or to show readers your familiarity with arcane works.

If a large background literature exists, consider referring readers to one or two published reviews to which they can refer rather than citing large numbers of individual works. You are writing for a professional audience; you may safely assume that most readers will be familiar with the general background literature and that they will only want to read about literature that is directly related to your rationale, method, or conclusions.

The Closing: Telling the Plan

After you have stated the rationale and set the background, it's time to bring the introduction to a close with a statement of purpose. Plan to get this done in one or two short to medium-length paragraphs

that specify the plan for your research (the variables manipulated, the hypotheses or research questions evaluated, the results expected). Statements of purpose typically begin with phrases such as

- *This study was designed to determine . . .*
- *In this study, I addressed the following questions . . .*
- *The purpose of this investigation was to explore . . .*
- *This report describes a controlled study of . . .*

Statements of purpose may be organized by questions or hypotheses:

- *The research described herein was designed to answer the following questions . . .*
- *Several questions were addressed in the research reported here . . .*

The statement of purpose may be phrased in terms of hypotheses to be evaluated:

- *In this study, we evaluated the following hypotheses . . .*
- *The findings of previous research suggest several hypotheses . . .*

Regardless of the format you choose, clearly identify the statement of purpose at the beginning of the paragraph before you elaborate on what it is.

Keeping Readers With You

Busy readers often decide within the first few sentences whether to continue reading an article. The first sentences you write may be the last sentences a reader reads if they are difficult to comprehend or do not appeal to the reader's interests. Mediocre writing later in a paper may sneak by, but if readers are confronted with poor writing in the introduction, they will be inclined to put your article aside and move on to something else. Your introduction is bait in an ocean of hungry readers, so make it as attractive as possible to catch the eye of your audience.

The introduction to your article is an introduction to the research you did, but it also is your introduction to your audience. As they read the introduction, readers are making judgments about your writing style, your ability to communicate, your ability to think logically, your ability to identify and solve problems, and your competence and trustworthiness. If your introduction is sloppy, disjointed, or difficult to follow, readers may conclude that your work cannot be taken seriously.

Guidelines for Writing the Introduction

- Work from the general (topic statement) to the specific (research questions).
- Identify the topic area.
- Tell the reader where your study fits in.
- Give the reader pertinent background information.
- Write chronologically within topics.
- Write tactically: focus on the important information, not all the information available.
- State research questions and hypotheses in a statement of purpose at the end of the introduction.
- Be a good "conversational partner": keep the reader interested in what you are saying.

References

Gamer, M., & Hecht, H. (2007). Are you looking at me? Measuring the cone of gaze. *Journal of Experimental Psychology: Human Perception and Performance, 33,* 705–715.

Guilmette, T. J., Temple, R. O., Kennedy, M. L., Weiler, M. D., Ruffolo, L. F., & Dufresne, E. (2005). The influence of victim characteristics on potential jurors' perceptions of brain damage in mild traumatic brain injury. *Brain Injury, 19,* 1027–1030.

Kane, T. (1988). *The new Oxford guide to writing* (p. 46). New York, NY: Oxford University Press.

Martin, E., & McDonald, S. (2005). Evaluating the causes of impaired irony comprehension following traumatic brain injury. *Aphasiology, 19,* 712–730.

Martinussen, R., & Tannock, R. (2006). Working memory impairments in children with attention-deficit hyperactivity disorder with and without comorbid language learning disorders. *Journal of Clinical and Experimental Neuropsychology, 28,* 1073–1094.

Moberg, C. A., & Curtin, J. J. (2009). Alcohol selectively reduces anxiety but not fear: Startle response to predictable versus unpredictable threat. *Journal of Abnormal Psychology, 118,* 335–347.

Shi, L-F. (2015). How "proficient" is proficient? Bilingual listeners' recognition of English words in noise. *American Journal of Audiology, 24,* 53–65.

Sternberg, R. J. (1993). How to win acceptances by psychology journals: 21 tips for better writing. *APS Observer.* Washington, DC: Association for Psychological Science.

Stolwyk, R. J., Charlton, J. L., Triggs, T. J., Iansek, R., & Bradshaw, J. L. (2006). Neuropsychological function and driving ability in people with Parkinson's disease. *Journal of Clinical and Experimental Neuropsychology, 28,* 898–913.

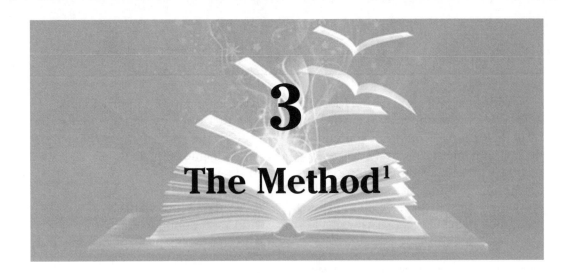

3

The Method[1]

"Though this be madness, yet there is method in't."

—William Shakespeare, *Hamlet, Act II, Scene 2*

The method section of a research article sets the stage for the presentation of findings in the results section. It describes the source of the data (the participants), the materials, the apparatus, and the procedures used to collect the data.

Information in the method section serves two primary purposes: it enables readers to judge the validity of the research, and it enables replication of your work by others. To convince readers of the internal validity of your work, you must show that your materials, apparatus, and procedures were appropriate to the research questions addressed and were sufficiently controlled to ensure that the independent variables were the only source of change in the dependent variables. To convince readers of the external validity of your work, you must show that your results are generalizable to other participants in other places and at other times. To permit others to replicate your work, you must provide enough information that a competent investigator with knowledge of the research area can duplicate the essential elements of your work.

Although you must include enough information in the method section for readers to judge and replicate your work, don't burden the reader with unnecessary detail. Specify only elements of the method that may affect your results or conclusions. Don't elaborate on normal practice, and don't include incidental details such as room temperature or lighting unless they are likely to affect participants' performances.

Organization of the Method Section

The method section of research articles in medical and behavioral science journals typically is divided into four subsections, each with its own heading:

- Participants (subjects)[2]
- Materials
- Apparatus
- Procedures

---

[1]The examples in this chapter, and the citations within them, are fictitious.
[2]When animals are the object of study, most contemporary journals refer to them as subjects. When humans are the object of study, most contemporary journals refer to them as participants.

Additional subsections may also be appropriate, depending on the complexity of the research. Complex experimental designs may merit a separate design subsection. Complex or unusual procedures for coding, scoring, data analysis, data reduction, or statistical evaluation may merit their own subsections as well.

Participants

The participants section of a research paper usually is a mix of identification (who the participants were) and procedures (how the participants were selected). The description of participants should accomplish two basic purposes: it should show that the participants are representative of the population to which the results are to be generalized, and it should provide enough information that a competent investigator can assemble a group that matches the study group on characteristics that may affect the results obtained. The description of participants typically includes

- how many were in the study;
- the population from which they were selected;
- how they were selected (e.g., random selection, stratified sampling, etc.);
- the number assigned to each condition or group and the procedures used to assign them;
- inducements used to recruit participants (e.g., compensation, course credit, contribution to knowledge); and
- verification that informed consent for participation was obtained (if the journal requires a statement in the paper itself).

The description of participants also should describe any characteristics that may affect the results. These characteristics often include

- age, sex, and education;
- racial or ethnic status;
- socioeconomic status;
- perceptual status (e.g., hearing and visual acuity);
- scores on screening tests; and
- demographic characteristics used to select participants (e.g., education level, medical diagnosis, presence of neuropathology).

If a characteristic is an experimental variable or might affect the results, describe it. If a characteristic may affect the extent to which your results apply to a population, describe it. If a characteristic helps readers get a better sense of your sample, describe it, even though it may not directly affect your results.

How much detail you provide about participants depends primarily on the uniqueness of the population to which you intend to generalize your findings. If you intend to generalize your findings to a typical population with few unique characteristics, a brief description of participants may suffice.

The participants were 1,000 adult residents of Metro City, Indiana, randomly selected from the 487,349 residents listed in the Metro City telephone directory. They ranged in age from 20 to 88. Half were male and half were female. The proportions of male and female participants were approximately equal (±3%) across age deciles from age 20 to age 90. The proportion of males and females within any age decile did not differ by more than 2%.

If the participants represent a special population, a more detailed description may be necessary. (Note the combination of identification and procedures in the following example.)

Twenty non-brain-injured adults and 20 adults with traumatic brain injuries participated in the experiment. Non-brain-injured participants ranged in age from 20 to 44 years of age, and had from 12 to 15 years of education. They were recruited by means of personal interviews from randomly selected students in the Business Administration program at Metropolitan Community College. Non-brain-injured participants reported no history of head injury, loss of consciousness, or neurologic complaints. Informed consent was obtained from each non-brain-injured participant. Each non-brain-injured participant scored less than 30 on the Minnesota Test for Detection of Brain Injury (MTDBI; Bibby & Vland, 1998). (MTDBI scores of 40 or below are considered to signify absence of brain injury.) Table 2 provides participant-by-participant ages, education levels, and MTDBI scores for non-brain-injured participants.

Brain-injured participants (30 M, 10 F) were randomly selected from a group of 132 brain-injured adults enrolled in rehabilitation programs at Gotham City Rehabilitation Center. Brain-injured participants ranged in age from 20 to 43 years and had completed from 11 to 16 years of education. At entry into the study each brain-injured participant was within 3 months post onset of a single closed-head injury and scored between 60 and 89 on the MTDBI.

None had experienced postinjury loss of consciousness exceeding 8 hours. A board-certified neuroradiologist estimated the site and extent of each brain-injured participant's brain injury from CT and MRI scans. Each brain-injured participant was tested with the Baranov Test of Cognitive Abilities (BTCA; Baranov & Chekov, 1999) and the Montgomery Memory Assessment (MMA: Montgomery and Ward, 1987). Informed consent for each brain-injured participant's inclusion in the study was obtained from the participant and the participant's next-of-kin or legal representative. Table 2 provides participant-by-participant ages, education levels, MTDBI scores, durations of coma, lesion sites, lesion extents, and scores on the BTCA and MMA for brain-injured participants.

If procedures used to select, screen, or recruit participants are complex, consider placing your description of the selection procedures under a separate heading. Here is an example of how elaborate participant identification, selection, and recruitment procedures might be set off from surrounding text by a heading.

Identification and Selection of Participants
Participants were 50 second-grade and 50 third-grade students from schools in Beadle County, South Dakota Unified School District 532. Participants were identified by their homeroom teachers who used a checklist of 16 behaviors known to be associated with auditory-visual integration disorder (AVID; Barney & Orlando, 2002). The 16 behaviors on the list are given in the Appendix. The parents of every student who exhibited 8 or more of

the 16 behaviors were sent a letter describing the research program and asking them to consent to their child's participation. Each parent who agreed attended a small-group session in which the objectives and procedures of the program were explained by the investigators. At the end of each small-group session, parents were given informed-consent forms, their questions were answered, and parents who wished their child to participate in the project were invited to sign the consent form . . .

Here is an example in which descriptions of screening tests used to select participants are set off with headings.

Screening Tests
Prior to entry into the study, participants were tested with a battery of screening tests to ensure adequate visual and auditory acuity to perceive task stimuli and to ensure that attentional impairments would not interfere with their performance of the experimental tasks.

Visual Acuity
Each participant was shown a white 125-by-200-mm card on which was printed a list of 20 bisyllabic words in 10-point Times New Roman typeface. Each word in the list was at or below sixth-grade reading level. A participant had to correctly read aloud at least 17 of the 20 words to qualify for inclusion in the study.

Auditory Acuity
Participants were required to pass a hearing screening at 1000 Hz, 2000 Hz, and 4000 Hz at 25 dB HL in order to participate in the study.

Attention
Each participant completed the Very Brief Test of Attention (VBTA; Cavanaugh & Castor, 2001), a computerized vigilance test. A participant had to score at least 80 on the VBTA to qualify for inclusion in the study. (VBTA scores above 70 are considered within the normal range.)

Materials

Experiments in the behavioral sciences often involve materials such as word lists, rating scales, questionnaires, and tests. If you need more than a few sentences to describe them, consider separating them from adjoining text with a heading. If your materials are complex, you might give an example, but if the example takes up a lot of space, put it in an appendix.

Description of materials usually precedes description of apparatus, because the materials typically are developed before the apparatus is assembled, and because the primary function of apparatus is to present the materials. The characteristics of the materials often define independent variables, so it may make sense to put the focus on the materials by describing them before describing the apparatus. If, however, readers' comprehension of what you write about your materials depends on their knowledge of the apparatus used to present them, describe the apparatus first, or incorporate a description of the apparatus into the description of materials.

Materials
Stimulus materials consisted of 12 gender-biased pictures and 12 neutral pictures. The gender-biased pictures

were colored line drawings showing an adult performing familiar daily activities that are characteristically thought of as either male or female oriented. (For example, a male-oriented picture showed a man painting a house; a female-oriented picture showed a woman removing clothing from a washing machine.) Six gender-biased pictures portrayed male-oriented activities, and six portrayed female-oriented activities. The 12 neutral pictures showed men or women performing activities with no appreciable gender bias (e.g., driving an automobile, walking a dog).

To confirm the gender bias of pictures, 20 female judges and 20 male judges were recruited from students enrolled in introductory psychology classes at Cirrus University. Groups of five students judged the gender bias of the pictures in rating sessions led by the investigator. Each judge was given a rating sheet on which were printed 24 seven-point scales numbered from 1 to 24. The seven points on each scale were labeled, from left to right, extreme male bias, moderate male bias, weak male bias, no bias, weak female bias, moderate female bias, and extreme female bias.

The judges were instructed in the procedures to be used in the rating session. The 24 pictures, each identified by number in the lower right corner, were projected on a screen in random order. Each picture remained on the screen for 1 min. The judges rated each picture's gender bias by circling a rating on the scale whose number matched the picture number.

Chronological order is commonly used to organize the description of materials, as in the next example that describes materials for a fictional experiment involving comprehension of spoken stories. The first section describes construction of the stories and the questions used to test comprehension of the stories. The second section describes how the stories and questions were later read aloud and recorded. (Note that the description of materials also includes description of procedures and apparatus. Such mixing of information relating to materials, the procedures used to produce the materials, and the apparatus used to record or present the materials is common in research papers.)

Materials
Stories and Questions
Ten test stories and two practice stories describing humorous situations familiar to adults in the United States were written for the experiment. The stories were controlled for number of words, average sentence length, and reading grade level. Reading grade levels were measured with the Cameron Readability Formula (Cameron, 1998). All stories were between Grade 5.2 and Grade 6.5 in reading difficulty. The practice stories averaged 150 words in length and ranged from 146 to 154 words long. The test stories averaged 200 words in length and ranged from 192 to 208 words long. Each test story contained 19 sentences and 54 non-repeated propositions. (See the Appendix for a sample test story.)

Eight yes/no questions were written for each story. Two tested stated main ideas, two tested implied main ideas, two tested stated details, and two tested implied details. Main idea questions tested central information that was repeated or elaborated on by other information in the story. Detailed questions tested peripheral information *that was mentioned only once and not elaborated on by other information in the story. Stated-information questions tested information that appeared in the story in the same form in which it subsequently was questioned. Implied-information questions tested information that was not directly stated but had to be inferred from other information in the story. The reading grade level of the questions ranged from Grade 4.9 to Grade 6.1. The questions were simple interrogatives and ranged from 9 to 12 words long. The procedures used to construct the questions and to determine that the questions actually tested stated and implied main ideas and details have been described elsewhere (Andover & Crosslink, 1999).*

Recording the Stories and Questions
The 12 stories and their questions were tape recorded as they were read aloud by a male native speaker of English who was trained to control the rate at which he read the stories. The speech rate for the stories ranged from 180 to 200 words per minute (Mean = 194 wpm). When the speaker finished reading each story, he paused for 5 s, said, "Here are the questions about this story," and, after a 4-s pause, read each question for the story, pausing for 20 s between questions. The stories and questions were recorded in a sound-attenuating chamber on Dynatech XLR audiotape via a Dynavoice XP300 microphone connected to an Audio Scientific 3500 audiotape deck.

The 12 tape-recorded stories were then copied to a Verbatim VF700 compact disc (CD) by means of an Audio Research 1200 sound card installed in a Paradox 8700 personal computer. The stories on the original CD were then copied to create five test CDs, each of which contained the two practice stories, in the same order, followed by a different random order of the 10 test stories. Each test CD was randomly assigned to four of the 20 participants in each group.

Sometimes other descriptive labels can be substituted for Materials. Stimuli may be used to signify materials such as sounds, symbols, words, or pictures, as in the following two examples.

Stimuli
Two 36-item sets of drawings and one 36-item set of photographs, each set representing 36 high-frequency picturable nouns, served as stimuli in the confrontation naming task. In one set of drawings, the nouns were depicted as black-and-white line drawings. In the other set of drawings, they were depicted as colored line drawings. In the photographs, the nouns were shown in color against a neutral gray background. The nouns represented in the drawings and pictures were within the first 5,000 most frequent English words listed in the New World Word Frequency Corpus (Sands & Gravell, 2000).

Stimuli
Stimuli were 48 nonsense words. Sixteen contained two syllables (e.g., lanim), 16 contained three syllables (e.g., mirafon), and 16 contained four syllables (e.g., tazarubir). The nonsense words were read aloud from a randomized list by a female native speaker of English who was trained to maintain standard English timing and stress patterns within words.

The speaker placed emphatic stress on the first syllable of two-syllable and three-syllable words and the third syllable of four-syllable words.

Tests may be the label of choice for materials such as standardized or non-standardized tests, including screening tests and tests used to assign participants to conditions, as in the following example. (Note the switch from passive voice to active voice in the second paragraph. It seems to us that active voice works well there, whereas passive voice reads more smoothly in the other paragraphs.)

Tests
To establish baseline reading levels, three tests of literacy skills (Hazen & Carlyle, 2002) were administered to participants before their entry into the reading program.

The Phoneme Segmentation Test assessed a child's ability to identify and produce individual sounds in three- and four-phoneme words. The examiner said a test word (e.g., "bat") and asked the child to say the phonemes in the word in the order they occurred in the word (e.g., "/b/ /æ/ /t/").

The Nonsense Word Test assessed a child's knowledge of letter-to-sound correspondence and sound-blending ability. The child was shown a page of vowel-consonant or consonant-vowel-consonant nonsense words and was asked to say the sounds one by one and then to say the nonsense word.

The Oral Reading Test assessed a child's fluency and accuracy when reading printed text. The child was shown a printed passage and asked to read it aloud. The child was told to stop reading after 1 min.

If your materials have been published elsewhere or have been adequately described in other work, provide a general description of the materials and refer readers to the other work, but describe the materials well enough to show readers that you have controlled characteristics that may affect participants' performance.

Stimuli
The words shown to participants in the lexical-decision task were randomly selected from Byron and Thackeray's (1994) list of words ranked by frequency in English and by subjective familiarity to English-speaking adults. Byron and Thackeray's rating scale ranged from 0 ("I have never seen or heard this word.") to 10 ("I see or hear this word every day.") All words were nouns, within the five million most frequent English words, and had familiarity ratings from 6 to 10 in Byron and Thackeray's list.

The materials section should be complete in itself. Do not force readers to find and read a source article to judge the adequacy and appropriateness of your materials, and do not refer readers to unpublished work or to works published in limited circulation, which are unlikely to be readily accessible.

Be careful not to overwhelm readers with inconsequential details. The description of materials should show readers that you have controlled characteristics that may affect the data you collect, but do not burden the materials section with information that has no bearing on interpretation of your findings. Readers can be an impatient lot. Give them too much to digest, and they will leave your table.

Apparatus

The apparatus section tells readers about the equipment used in your research. When you describe the apparatus, try to give readers a mental image of the environment in which the research took place. Describe the components of the apparatus, how they were connected, and what they did in enough detail to permit readers to evaluate whether the apparatus was appropriately selected, designed, and used. Your description also should permit a person who replicates your work to assemble equivalent apparatus. (Equivalent does not mean identical. It means that differences between your equipment and that used in the replication do not affect the data obtained.)

The apparatus section often begins with a description of the surroundings in which an experiment takes place, as in the following example.

Participants were tested individually while sitting at a table in a quiet, dimly lighted testing room. The table faced the rear wall of the testing room. Two Laudenkloss 480 SL speakers were attached to the rear wall of the testing room, 24 inches above the tabletop and 30 inches on each side of the midline of the table. The speakers were connected to equipment in an adjoining control room. A one-way-vision window behind the participant permitted an observer in the control room to observe events in the testing room.

Mention but do not describe generic items of apparatus such as furniture, stopwatches, buzzers, and the like. Identify manufacturers and provide model numbers for commercially available equipment such as tape recorders, speakers, microphones, and personal computers. Custom-built equipment often requires elaborate description, as in this example.

A three-key response console was on the table in front of the participant. The response console consisted of an 8" L by 4" W by 2" D gray metal box on the top surface of which was a horizontal row of three 1-inch-square pushbuttons. The middle pushbutton was centered on the top surface of the box, and the left-side and right-side pushbuttons were set 2 inches on either side of the center. The pushbuttons were illuminated from below. The word "YES" was centered one-half inch below the left pushbutton, the words "DON'T KNOW" were centered one-half inch below the middle pushbutton, and the word "NO" was centered one-half inch below the right pushbutton. The words were printed in quarter-inch-high black letters on a white background. Activation of any pushbutton produced an electronic signal that uniquely identified it to other components of apparatus.

When you write the apparatus section, do not simply list apparatus items and describe how they are connected. Such lists are difficult for readers to comprehend and almost impossible to remember. Organize the apparatus section so that it tells readers how the components work together to perform their functions (e.g., present stimuli, control conditions, or record participants' responses). Group items of apparatus according to what they do. Describe functional groups by telling how they perform their function.

A Paradox 8700 personal computer was located in the control room. An Orion 450D compact disc (CD) drive and an

Audio Research 4750 sound card were installed in the computer. The sound card was connected to the inputs of an Audiotech 4900 amplifier in the control room. The speaker outputs of the amplifier were connected to the Laudenkloss speakers in the testing room so that CDs in the computer CD drive could be played through the speakers in the testing room. The signals from the pushbuttons on the response console in the testing room were sent to the personal computer via a Bantam 1280XP interface card.

A schematic may lessen readers' workload if the apparatus is complex. Figure 3–1 shows a schematic used to illustrate instrumentation used to gather biophysical measures in a study of stuttering. Each piece of apparatus in the figure should be described in the text as well.

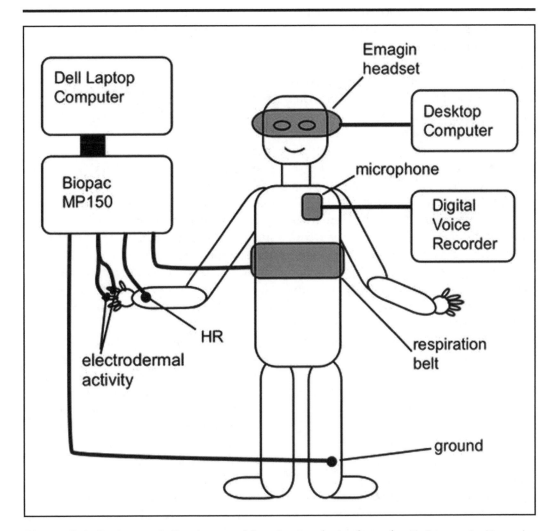

Figure 3–1. Instrumentation to record heart rate, electrodermal activity, respiration rate, and speech samples.

When your reader has a clear mental picture of your materials and knows what your apparatus was and what it did, you are ready to tell the reader what happened to participants during data collection. You do this in the procedures section.

Procedures

The procedures section is best arranged chronologically. Describe, in the order in which they occurred, important characteristics of the procedure, but do not describe in detail well-known standard procedures such as administration of standardized tests or collection of personal information. The procedures section should contain enough information for informed readers to judge the adequacy and appropriateness of the procedures, and should describe participants, materials, and procedures so that a trained investigator can replicate the study, but no more.

Participants are often given instructions before experimental tasks or treatments begin. If you instruct participants, provide the gist of the instructions. Do not include verbatim transcripts. Most readers are familiar with standard instructional procedures and don't need to know their exact content. A few sentences describing their general form usually are enough, unless the instructions are themselves an experimental variable or are likely to affect the outcome of the study.

Each participant was seated at the table in the testing room. The experimenter told each participant that he or she would hear several stories, and after each story the participant would hear several questions about the story that could be answered

"yes," "no," or "don't know," by pressing the appropriate button on the response console. The experimenter answered the participant's questions, if any were asked. When a participant indicated that he or she understood the instructions, the experimenter played the practice stories from the test CD assigned to that participant. The experimenter provided instruction, demonstration, replayed the practice stories, and answered questions as needed until he was confident that the participant understood the requirements of the task.

Design

If the design of your experiment is complex, you can lessen readers' workload with a design section in which you describe the independent variables (conditions, groups) and dependent variables (measures), tell how participants were selected and assigned to groups, and describe other important general features of the method. Here is an example of a design section for a study of reading comprehension.

This experiment employed a repeated-measures design with three between-conditions variables and two between-participants variables. The between-conditions variables were speaker (male versus female), directness (stated information versus implied information), and salience (main ideas versus details). The within-participants variables were age (20 to 49 years versus 50 to 79 years) and reading level (Grades 6 through 9 versus Grades 10 through 14).

Here is a sample of a design section for a single-subject study of conversational behavior. It combines description of the design with related aspects of procedure.

A single-subject multiple-baseline design was employed to assess participants' use of three pragmatic conversational behaviors during baseline, treatment, and maintenance phases. During the baseline phase, the frequency and appropriateness of turn-taking, topic changing, and conversational repair were measured. During the first phase of treatment, one behavior was trained and the other two behaviors periodically were measured to assess potential generalization of training effects (generalization probes). When the frequency and appropriateness of the first trained behavior reached criterion, treatment was applied to the second behavior, while the third behavior was periodically measured to assess generalization, and the first behavior was periodically measured to assess maintenance (maintenance probes).

Data Collection (Data Acquisition)

When data-collection procedures are complex, important, or unusual, describe them in a separate section, as in the two examples that follow.

Data Collection
A customized software program installed in the personal computer accumulated response data from each participant. The software program
matched each press of a pushbutton by a participant with the test story and question that preceded the pushbutton press. The program then accumulated in a database a record of each participant's correct and incorrect responses to each of the four question types (stated main idea, implied main idea, stated detail, implied detail) for each story.

Data Acquisition
The signals from the microphone were amplified (Electrotech Model PA 4640), low-pass filtered at 8 kHz (Electrotech Model SF 4210), and recorded on a digital tape recorder (General Acoustics Model DR 5450) at a sampling rate of 48 kHz. The signals from sensors on the lip, jaw, and larynx were digitized at 1 kHz per channel, converted to binary files, and exported to a Dataworks 7.3 data analysis program (Dataworks General, Bridgeton, CT) installed on the hard drive of a Genesis Model 1200 personal computer.

Data Coding and Scoring

When observers transcribe, code, or score information gathered during the data-collection phase of a study, the procedures used may be placed in separate sections of procedures, as in the following examples.

Transcription and Scoring
Each participant's spoken responses to the elicitation stimuli, together with any prompts delivered by the examiner, were recorded on audiotape. A speech-language pathologist familiar with the speech of brain-injured adults orthographically transcribed each speech sample. Then a second speech-

language pathologist independently transcribed the speech samples. When the two disagreed on how a speech event should be transcribed, a third speech-language pathologist reviewed the event in question, and the three reached a consensus decision on how the event should be transcribed. Then the speech samples were scored for the presence of speech deviations using published rules (Adams & Evenson, 2005).

Categorization of Speech Behaviors
Speech behaviors that qualified as words and were accurate and informative relative to an eliciting stimulus were scored as correct information units. Speech behaviors that qualified as words but were not informative were assigned to one of six categories: inaccurate word, false start, exact repetition, nonspecific word, filler word, or irrelevant word. Speech behaviors that did not qualify as words were assigned to one of three categories: unintelligible, part-word, or non-word filler.

Reliability

When data are based on subjective decisions made by observers (e.g., assigning behaviors to categories, recording the occurrence of certain behaviors, rating aspects of performance), most journals require that the reliability of the decisions be reported, often in a separate section, as in the following example.

Reliability
To assess interjudge agreement for scoring performance deviations, a

graduate student with training in the scoring system independently scored transcripts for eight randomly selected participants from the control group and eight randomly selected participants from the treatment group. Point-to-point interjudge agreement between the original scoring and the second scoring was 85% or greater for each of the nine performance deviation categories. The interjudge agreement for scoring words and informative words has been reported previously (Conrad & Penfield, 2003) and exceeded 90% point-to-point agreement for each of 20 speech samples.

Statistical Analysis

Sometimes authors provide a separate section describing statistical methods used to analyze results, usually when the statistical methods are complex or not well known. However, unless statistical analyses are complex or employ procedures that are not widely known, it usually is more efficient to describe the analyses when you present the results.

Statistical Models
Bates' proportional risk estimates (Bates, 1998) were calculated to identify independent predictors of dementia risk in late life. The proportional risk model is commonly used in survival analysis and medical testing studies. The model assumes that changing the value of stressors (explanatory variables) multiplies risk by a constant amount for each stressor. The cumulative effects of the changes in stressor values allow the risk for a given individual to be estimated. In

this study, two risk factor models were calculated for each stress variable—an unadjusted model and a model adjusted for age at initial diagnosis of dementia. Stressor variables entered into both models were hypertension, diabetes, elevated cholesterol, and smoking.

Style

Write the method section in past tense, because you are describing activities that took place in the past. Make liberal use of passive voice. Passive voice works well in the method section because the focus is on actions and not agents, and because the identity of agents is implied and unimportant. Method sections written in active voice tend to be stilted and repetitious. Don't, however, feel compelled to use only passive voice in the method section. Long strings of sentences written in passive voice can be tiring, so look for places where you can drop in an active-voice sentence to break the monotony.

> *The 20 participants came from freshman English classes at Adams University (active). Each participant was paid $50 (passive). The Franklin Aptitude Test was administered to each participant (passive). The 10 with the lowest scores made up an instruction group, and the 10 with the highest scores made up a no-instruction group (active).*

Don't shun passive sentences in the method section. But don't overdo them. Too many sentences of the same form, whether active or passive, quickly lead to monotony. Choose active or passive voice intentionally, based on the focus and continuity of what you are trying to communicate. (*See* also Passive Voice later in this book in Chapter 12: Copy Editing for more on passive voice in science writing.)

Guidelines for Writing the Method

- Tell the reader who (participants) did what (procedures) and what they used (materials, apparatus) to do it.
- Imagine you were trying to replicate your study. What would you want to know? Write that.
- Organize the apparatus section so that it tells readers how the components work together to perform their functions (e.g., present stimuli, control conditions, or record participants' responses).
- Describe, in the order in which they occurred, important characteristics of the procedure.
- Write the method section in past tense, because you are describing activities that took place in the past, but look for places where you can drop in an active-voice sentence to break the monotony.

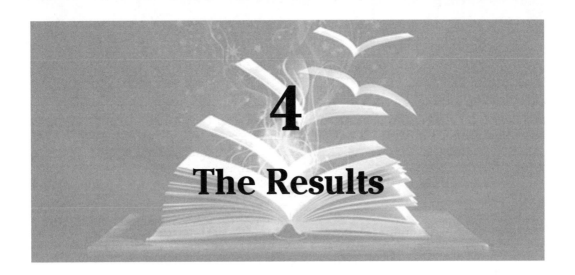

4
The Results

"All we want are the facts, ma'am."
—Jack Webb, Dragnet

The purpose of the results section is to present the findings of your study. Keep your writing simple and direct. Results sections may seem "stilted" and redundant (we found this, and then we found this, and then this), but that's OK. There are standard ways to present results of statistical analyses; follow the rules discussed below. Resist the urge to make the results section read like a novel. Your results are not a fictional work; do not make the reader wait to find out what you found. Unlike a mystery novel, start the results section with "the big reveal" of your main finding. Keep thoughts about what the findings mean for the discussion section. Readers are expecting to find a summary of your data and the results of the statistical analyses completed. In fact, this is a good way to organize the results section.

Most results sections start by directing the reader's attention to a table that provides a summary of your data. You have collected a lot of data; there is no way to present every data point to the reader, and doing so would be tedious and difficult to follow. Instead, provide a summary that includes measures of central tendency and measures of variability for each of your findings. Measures of central tendency and variability are sometimes called "descriptive statistics," because they give the reader a brief description of your data without having to present all of it. The exact nature of these measures depends on the types of dependent variables measured. The independent and dependent variables should be obvious from this table.

In Table 4–1, the independent variables are group (stuttering versus social phobia) and time of measurement (immediately after giving a speech versus 6 weeks later via video review). The dependent variables are self-ratings of speech naturalness and overall quality of the speech.

Commonly Used Statistics in Communication Sciences and Disorders

Researchers control independent variables and measure the independent variable's effects on dependent variables. Both the nature of the research question and the nature of the dependent variable determine the statistical tests used to evaluate the effects of the independent variable(s)

Table 4–1. Group Means (Standard Deviation) for Self-Ratings of Speech Naturalness and Overall Quality of Speech Obtained Immediately After Giving a Speech and 6 Weeks Later After Viewing the Same Videotaped Speech

	Group				
	Stuttering (*n* = 20)		Social Phobia (*n* = 20)		
Time of Measurement	Naturalness*	Overall Quality of Speech**	Naturalness	Overall Quality of Speech	
Immediately post speech	5.10 (1.89)	5.30 (2.16)	4.27 (1.03)	3.14 (0.65)	
Six weeks post video	6.83 (0.98)	6.33 (1.37)	6.00 (1.98)	5.69 (1.78)	

Note. *Speech naturalness was rated on a 1 to 9 scale, with 1 = "very unnatural" and 9 = "very natural." **Overall quality of speech was rated on a 1 to 9 scale, with 1 = "very low quality" and 9 = "very high quality."

on the dependent variable. Researchers might ask questions about possible differences between variables, or relationships between them, or seek to model how a number of variables influence one another. The statistical tests used for each of these types of questions are different, and therefore, the nature of the research question contributes to the decision regarding what statistic to use. The nature of the dependent variable (DV) is the other determinant. Some DVs are nominal (categories), some are ordinal (in an order), some are interval (in lockstep order), and some are ratio (a ratio!). When thinking about statistics, the most important distinctions are between nominal/ordinal versus interval/ratio. Nonparametric statistics are used for nominal and ordinal-level data, whereas parametric statistics are used for interval or ratio data. There is no one correct statistic to use in all instances. The nature of the research question and the nature of the dependent variable being measured determine what statistic is the correct one to use. So how do you decide if the statistics used were the correct ones? Nonparametric statistics are used when any one of the following occurs: the data are not normally distributed, the sample size is small, or the dependent variables are nominal or ordinal. Parametric statistics are used when data are normally distributed (like a bell curve shape), sample sizes are large, and the dependent variables are interval or ratio. Tables 4–2 and 4–3 give some examples of commonly used statistics in Communication Sciences and Disorders (CSD).

Special Cases

If the statistical analyses in your manuscript are new and/or uncommon, journal editors may ask you to add a section that explains the analyses in greater detail. Explain why you chose the statistic, state research questions that the new statistic answers that cannot be answered by more commonly used statistics, and define any new terms associated with the new statistic. If the test required transformation of

Table 4–2. Statistical Tests That Compare Differences Between Groups or Between Conditions Within a Group

Name of Test	Test Statistic	Dependent Variable Is	Number of Independent Variables	Number of Dependent Variables	Example
Nonparametric					
Chi-square	χ^2	Nominal			IV: Gender (Male versus Female)
					DV: Appropriateness of pitch (yes or no)
Mann-Whitney	U	Ordinal or small n	1	1	IV: Gender (Male versus Female)
					DV: high, medium, or low pitch rating
Wilcoxon Signed-Ranks Test	W_x	Ordinal or small n	1	1	IV: Gender (Male versus Female versus MtF)
					DV: high, medium, or low pitch
Kruskal-Wallis one-way ANOVA	KW	Ordinal or small n	1 (with >2 levels)	1	IV: Gender (Male versus Female versus MtF)
					DV: low, middle, or high pitch rating
Friedman two-way ANOVA by ranks	F_r	Ordinal or small n	2	1	IVs: Gender (Male versus Female) *and* Age (child versus adult)
					DV: low, middle, or high pitch
Parametric					
t-test	t	Interval or ratio	1	1	IV: Gender (Male versus Female)
					DV: F_0
One-way ANOVA	F	Interval or ratio	1 (with >2 levels)	1	IV: Gender (Male versus Female versus MtF)
					DV: F_0

continues

Table 4–2. *continued*

Name of Test	Test Statistic	Dependent Variable Is	Number of Independent Variables	Number of Dependent Variables	Example
Two-way ANOVA	*F*	Interval or ratio	2	1	IVs: Gender (Male versus Female) *and* Age (child versus adult) DV: F_0
Three-way ANOVA	*F*	Interval or ratio	3	1	IVs: Gender *and* Age *and* Race (African American versus Caucasian) DV: F_0
MANOVA	*F*	Interval or ratio	1	Two or more	IV: Gender (Male versus Female versus MtF) DVs: F_0, F_2 (resonance)

Note. *IV* = independent variable, *DV* = dependent variable, *MtF* = male to female transgender person.

Table 4–3. Statistics Addressing Relationships

Name of Test	Test Statistic	Dependent Variable Is	Example
Nonparametric			
Spearman	*rho*	Ordinal or small *n*	Is there a relationship between stuttering severity (mild, moderate, severe) and audience size?
Parametric			
Pearson Product Moment Correlation	*r*	Interval or ratio	Is there a correlation between the percentage of stuttered syllables (%SS) and the size of an audience?
Regression			What aspects of an audience predict %SS? Size of audience? Gender? Attentiveness?

the data, report the nature of these transformations and how they were done. Refer the reader to other work that described or used the analyses, so that interested readers can learn more about it.

How to Report Statistics

Three numbers are required when reporting the results of parametric and nonparametric statistics: the alpha value (α) for significance, the number resulting from the statistical analysis (called the "test statistic"), and the probability value (p) associated with the analysis. Researchers set the alpha value prior to carrying out statistical analyses. By convention, alpha is typically set at .05 or lower, meaning that researchers are willing to be incorrect in their findings 5% of the time or less. Once alpha is set, it's time to calculate the test statistic and associated probability (p) value. For example, an analysis of variance (ANOVA) could be used to compare the performance of three groups of participants. The ANOVA yields a number (the F statistic) and an associated p-value for the comparisons between the three groups. The researcher then compares the p-value with the alpha value. If the p-value is less than the alpha value, then the results between groups are said to be "significantly different." If the p-value is greater than the alpha value, then the results are "not significantly different." Researchers should report the test statistic, alpha, and p-value for each analysis completed.

Additional numbers may be required, such as the effect size and the observed power. These numbers, along with sample size, are important because they help interpret the results. We will define each of these numbers and then explain how they are related.

Effect size refers to the magnitude of the difference between two means or the strength of the relationship between variables. Effect sizes are reported in standard deviation units; this allows comparison of results across variables, conditions, or studies. Effect sizes are used to compare the outcomes of treatment studies and are often used as indicators of "practical significance." For example, let's say you have two treatments and both have statistically significant increases in pre-post mean scores, but one has a larger effect size than the other. The treatment with the larger effect size has a bigger effect on outcome compared to the treatment with the smaller effect size.

Many metrics are available for reporting effect size; two of the more common metrics are Cohen's d and partial eta squared (η_p^2). Cohen was a statistician who published guidelines (Cohen, 1992) for interpreting d as small (generally 0.20 SD or less), medium (0.5 SD), or large (0.80 SD or above). Partial eta squared is the type of effect size reported by SPSS, a commonly used statistical software package. A η_p^2 of 0.01 is considered a small effect, 0.06 is considered a medium-sized effect, and 0.14 is considered a large effect (Clark-Carter, 1997, p. 254). The type of effect size reported depends on the statistics used.

Power refers to the ability to detect a difference between variables when one actually exists. Power ($1 - \beta$) ranges from 0 to 1. Unlike alpha, there is no conventional level of acceptance for power, although most researchers would aim for at least .80. Power is reported only when no significant differences are found; essentially, the researcher is saying, "I had enough power (.80 or above) to detect a difference if one was there, and because I did not find one, that means there is no true difference between these groups or variables."

Alpha, effect size, power, and sample size are related. With alpha set to .05, if the size of the effect between groups is small (small differences between groups), then you need more participants (larger sample size) in order to have enough power to see the small difference. Conversely, if the effect size is large, then fewer participants are necessary in order to have enough power to detect the large difference.

Statistics software will report all the required numbers described above. The publication manual of the American Psychological Association (American Psychological Association, 2010) stipulates formats to use for reporting the numbers. These formats are a "shorthand" for reporting the results of statistical tests. For example, you might see the following in a results section:

$$F\,(2,\,24) = 16.98,\, p = .02,\, \eta_p^2 = 0.18.$$

This tells us that the researchers used a parametric statistic (in this case ANOVA). They are reporting the test statistic associated with ANOVA (the "*F*") and the value of the test statistic (in this example, 16.98). Degrees of freedom are reported in parentheses following the *F*. Degrees of freedom (or *df*) are part of the statistical analyses and are related to the number of variables and comparisons present in the study. The next part is the *p*-value. The *p*-value is the probability value associated with the statistical analysis that was completed. The effect size calculation follows ("partial eta squared" or η_p^2); in this example, the effect is quite large. The only information "missing" from this shorthand report is the alpha value. Sometimes researchers will state the alpha value in their results section ("The alpha for significance was set at .01"). When left unstated, it is generally assumed that alpha equals .05.

The *r* is the test statistic for the Pearson Product Moment Correlation, a parametric statistic that assesses relationships among variables. The shorthand for reporting correlations looks a bit different:

$$r = -.90,\, p = .01.$$

The "−.90" is the value of the test statistic. The "*p* = .01" is the probability value associated with the statistical analysis that was completed. Correlations tell us about (a) the strength of the relationships among two or more variables, and (b) the direction of the relationships. Correlations can range from −1 to +1. Correlations that are close to zero indicate that there are not strong relationships between the variables being studied. The closer a correlation gets to either −1 or +1, the stronger the relationship is between the variables. The direction of the relationship is indicated by the +/− signs. Negative correlations indicate that as one variable increases, the other decreases. A "strong negative correlation" means that this relationship is systematic. For example, there are likely strong negative correlations between the amount of stuttering and speech naturalness scores (as stuttering frequency increases, naturalness decreases).

Writing the Results Section

It may help to have a copy of your research questions in front of you as you write your results; this will keep your writing focused and serves as a checklist to make sure you've answered each question.

Work From Broad to Narrow

After presenting your descriptive snapshot of your data, report the results of omnibus statistical tests for your main findings. Omnibus statistical tests evaluate main effects and possible interactions between the main effects. Main effects are comparisons of each independent variable (e.g., male versus female versus MtF; child versus adult; AA versus Caucasian in Table 4–2). A "significant main effect for gender" means that at least one of the gender comparisons (male versus female, male versus MtF, female versus

MtF) is significant. Notice that the omnibus test only tells you that at least one of these comparisons is significant; it does not tell you which one. Follow-up tests, sometimes called "pairwise comparisons" or "planned comparisons," are used to determine which comparisons are significant. The omnibus test also evaluates all possible interactions between variables (gender, age, race).

Report the results of the omnibus test and any follow-up tests, using the appropriate shorthand: name the test used, identify the comparison being addressed, and report the statistic and p-value you used to evaluate the comparison. Next, state if the result was significant or not. Then provide a brief statement of what the finding means. Repeat this general format for each omnibus test and follow-up procedures that you completed. Here are some examples:

An independent samples t-test was used to evaluate possible group differences in fundamental frequency ($t = 12.21$, $p = .001$). Results of this analysis indicate that there was a significant difference between groups in fundamental frequency. Review of the means of each group indicates that females had significantly higher fundamental frequency than did MtF participants.

Results of the 2 × 3 between-groups ANOVA revealed significant main effects for both the dysarthria group [$F(1, 195) = 32.75$, $p < .005$; $\eta_p^2 = .144$] and listening condition [$F(2, 195) = 16.54$, $p < .005$, $\eta_p^2 = .145$]. The interaction effect was not significant [$F(2, 195) = 2.87$, $p = .059$, $\eta_p^2 = .029$]. Planned comparisons revealed a significant difference between the topic knowledge (TK) and control conditions

($p < .005$). Intelligibility scores from the TK and familiarization conditions did not differ significantly ($p = .53$), indicating that both methods of training produced similar magnitudes of facilitative effects (Utianski, Lansford, Liss, & Azuma, 2011).

A series of repeated-measures ANOVA revealed significant main effects for directness $F(2, 38) = 6.45$, $p = .001$, salience $F(2, 38) = 12.93$, $p = .01$, and age $F(2, 38) = 8.35$, $p = .01$. The main effects for speaker gender $F(2, 38) = 0.41$, $p = .80$ and for reading level $F(2, 38) = 1.78$, $p = .06$ were not significant. There was a significant age by directness interaction $F(2, 38) = 10.67$, $p = .01$. Comprehension was better for stated ideas and for main ideas, and the younger participants had higher overall comprehension scores. Older participants had better comprehension for main ideas than details, whereas younger participants had equal levels of comprehension for main ideas and details.

Note that the above two examples differ in their use of brackets. Utianski et al. (2011) used brackets to enclose the statistical shorthand of their multiple comparisons. Although this is not technically correct per APA guidelines (APA, 2010), we think that the brackets make it easier to read than the second example above, without brackets.

When to Use Section Headings, Graphs, and Tables

Sometimes the research questions become headers in the results section. This can be helpful to readers, particularly if the questions are complex, but don't overdo it. Often the research questions can be shortened to more succinct headers, such as "between-group comparisons" or "within-group comparisons" or "correlational analyses." If all three comparisons are being reported, our preference is to report the between-group differences first, then the within-group comparisons, and finally correlational analyses.

The adage "a picture is worth a thousand words" is applicable to results sections. Think like a reader. If the results are easier to understand visually, then put those findings in a graph or figure. For example, in Figure 4–1, it would be misleading to report measures of central tendency in a table. Instead, showing the reader a picture of the data makes it immediately evident that the distribution is bimodal.

After reading the results section, readers know how you analyzed your data and what results you found. You have given them the facts. Now it's time to write the discussion, and tell them what those facts mean.

Guidelines for Writing the Results

- Have I answered all the research questions?
- Have I written from the general to the specific, starting with my biggest finding?
- Have I used standard reporting formats for my statistical analyses?

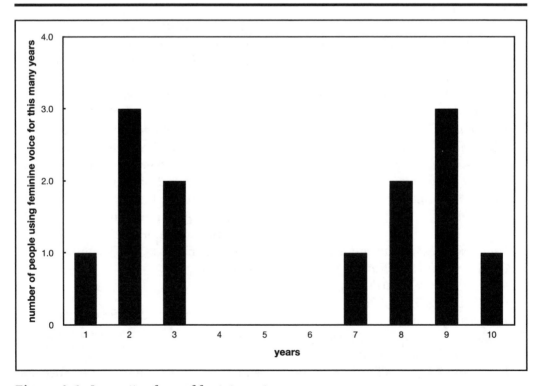

Figure 4–1. Longevity of use of feminine voice.

■ If my results were a fiction novel, does it read more like Ernest Hemingway and less like James Joyce?

References

American Psychological Association. (2010). *Publication manual of the American Psychological Association* (6th ed.). Washington, DC: Author.

Clark-Carter, D. (1997). *Doing quantitative psychological research: From design to report.* Hove, East Essex, UK: Psychology Press.

Cohen, J. (1992). A power primer. *Psychological Bulletin, 112,* 155–159.

Utianski, R., Lansford, K., Liss, J., & Azuma, T. (2011). The effects of topic knowledge on intelligibility and lexical segmentation in Hypokinetic and Ataxic dysarthria. *Journal of Medical Speech Language Pathology, 19,* 25–36.

5

Constructing Data Tables

"You can use all the quantitative data you can get, but you still have to distrust it and use your own intelligence and judgment."

—Alvin Toffler (Boone, 1999)

An investigator's intelligence and judgment play important parts in determining the character of the results presented in a research article. Intelligence enables the investigator to identify the important results. Judgment enables the investigator to organize the results in such a way that the important findings are conveyed clearly, concisely, and comprehensibly. Data tables are one way of reaching those goals.

Elements of Data Tables

A typical data table contains three major elements—a title, a body, and one or more table notes. The table title tells what the table is about. The table body contains headings and data cell entries. Table notes highlight important elements, identify units of measurement, specify important characteristics of the data, provide keys to abbreviations and symbols, elaborate on or qualify table entries, or indicate the results of statistical tests of significance.

Title

There is no universal format for table titles. Most journals require that titles begin with the word *Table* followed by an Arabic numeral and a period (e.g., Table 5.). Number tables in the order in which they are first mentioned in the text. Do not attach suffix letters to table numbers (e.g., Table 1a, Table 1b). If you want to add suffix letters because two tables contain related data, combine them into one table. (Tables in book chapters may be numbered according to the chapter in which they appear—e.g., the third table in Chapter 5 is Table 5–3).

Give every table a short but clear title in which key words orient readers to important elements of the table. Table titles usually are not complete sentences, as in the following examples:

- *Table 1. Brain-Injured Adults' Test Performance in Three Feedback Conditions.*
- *Table 1. Analysis of Variance for Recognition Scores.*

■ *Table 1. Reliability of Observers' Judgments of Fluency.*
■ *Table 1. Absorption Rates for Five Concentrations of Phosphate.*

Keep table titles concise. Include only enough information to enable the reader to get a sense of what is in the table without surrounding text. If you can use a general label for sets of data, do so. If the meanings of column or row headings would be obvious to readers, do not define them in the title.

Do not make the title a list of column heads and stubs.

Table 1. Performance of Groups Receiving Immediate Treatment, Delayed Treatment, or No Treatment on Posttreatment Tests of Speech Fluency, Listening Comprehension, and Reading Comprehension.

Instead, use general descriptors to group column heads and stubs.

Table 1. Performance of Groups on Language Tests.

Do not be so vague that the table can be about almost anything.

Table 1. Aggressive Behaviors.

Instead, give enough information to tell readers specifically what the table is about.

Table 1. Number of Aggressive Behaviors Observed During Time-Out From Reinforcement.

Here are a few examples of too-general, too-detailed, and about-right table titles.

Too general: *Reaction Times.*

Too detailed: *Mean Reaction Times (In Ms) for 20 Clinically Depressed Adults in Immediate Feedback, Delayed Feedback, and No Feedback Conditions.*

About right: *Reaction Times (in ms) for Clinically Depressed Adults in Three Feedback Conditions.*

Too general: *Whatsit Memory Test Scores.*

Too detailed: *Means, Standard Deviations, And Ranges for Whatsit Memory Test Scores of Young, Middle-Aged, and Old Male and Female Adult Participants.*

About right: *Age, Gender, and Whatsit Memory Test Scores.*

General information about a table or entries in a table may be given in the title.

Table 1. Regional Migration: 1990–2003 (rounded to nearest one hundred thousand).

Table 1. Medical Facility Visits by Young or Old Men and Women (n = 50 per group).

Table 1. Growth in Industrial Production from 1950 to 2000 (in 1950 dollars).

Sometimes information about table entries may be added to the title as a separate comment.

Table 1. Prevalence of Obesity in the United States, 1990–2002. (Obesity = body mass index [BMI] of 30 or greater.)

Table 1. Health Insurance Coverage and Number of Doctor Visits by Age and Sex. (From U.S. Department of Public Health Centers for Disease Control Report 2002–41, 2002.)

Do not cram too many comments into a table title. If the title contains more than two or three short comments, consider moving some to a table note.

Some style manuals require capitalization of all major words in table titles. Others require capitalization only of the first word in a title, plus proper nouns and acronyms. Some require that all words in a title be italicized. Others restrict italics to technical terms. Almost all journals require that tables in submitted manuscripts be double spaced, including titles and notes. Look at the information for authors on the journal's website or read the publishers' style manual for detailed guidance.

Notes

Table notes are lines of text placed below the body of a table. Table notes provide a place to add explanatory or qualifying information when the information would be too long, too obtrusive, or too distracting in the title. Notes may explain abbreviations and symbols, qualify or elaborate on table elements, specify sources of data, cite permissions, or indicate the significance of statistical findings. Table notes fall into three categories.

General notes apply to the table as a whole. A general note may specify important aspects of the data in a table, as in Table 5–1.

A general note may give the source of information in a table, as in Table 5–2.

A general note may provide keys to abbreviations and symbols in a table, as in Table 5–3.

Specific notes apply to a particular row, column, or entry. Several different systems for identifying specific notes are used in journals. Some use superscript letters or numerals. Others use standard footnote symbols ($\P$, $\S$, $\dagger$, $\ddagger$).

A specific note may elaborate on a column or row heading, as in Table 5–4.

Table 5–1. Example of a General Note in a Table

Score	87	129	111	97	103	73

Note. Scores on the *Whatsit Memory Test* may range from 0 to 140.

Table 5–2. Example of a Table Note Identifying Sources of Information

Score	87	129	111	97	103	73

Source: From K. K. Battles & V. Y. Catlin. (1998). A new test for assessing memory in normal adults and adults with dementia. *Journal of Memory, 55,* 102–123. Copyright 1998 by the Academy of Memory Science. Reprinted with permission.

Table 5–3. Defining Abbreviations in a Table Note

Score	87	129	111	97	103	73

Note. *SMTM* = Short-term Memory Test, *SFS* = Syntactic Flexibility Scale.

A specific note may elaborate on or qualify a table entry or a group of table entries, as in Table 5–5.

Probability notes indicate the results of statistical tests of significance. Most journals use asterisks to denote probability levels, as in Table 5–6.

Some journals use combinations of asterisks and daggers:

* $p < .05$ one-tailed
** $p < .01$ one-tailed
† $p < .05$ two-tailed
‡ $p < .01$ two-tailed

There is no universal format for table notes, but most journals require that general notes be placed first, specific notes second, and probability notes third. Consult the publisher's style manual or the journal's website to determine which format to use. Here are the conventions prescribed by the American Psychological Association, whose style recommendations are followed by many publications in the social and behavioral sciences.

General Note

Begin a general note at the left margin with the word *Note* (capitalized and italicized) followed by a period, and continue with the first general note on the same line. If there are multiple general notes, type them in succession without line breaks between notes.

Table 5–4. Example of a Specific Table Note

Group	Number*	Pretest	Posttest
Coaching	18	49.3	76.5
—	—	—	—

Note. *Number: number who completed at least 10 treatment sessions.

Table 5–5. Example of a Specific Table Note

Participant	Age	Education	Score
P1	56	12	48.7*
—	—	—	—

Note. *The mean score for this participant is based on 98 responses.

Table 5–6. Example of a Probability Table Note

Group	Pretest	Posttest	Difference
Coaching	46.9	63.2	16.3*
Support	47.3	86.4	39.1**
—	—	—	—

Note. *$p < .05$; **$p < .01$.

Specific Note

Show the within-table reference point for a specific note by placing a superscript lowercase letter (e.g., [a, b, c]) at the reference point in the table for each specific note. Begin each specific note at the left margin with the appropriate superscript letter, followed by the body of the note. If there are multiple specific notes, type them in succession with no line breaks between notes. Begin the specific notes for each table with the letter "a" (that is, do not use [a, b, c] in Table 1 and [c, d, e] in Table 2).

Probability Note

By convention, asterisks are used to signify the alpha level (Type 1 error level) of tests of significance. A single asterisk typically signifies alpha level $p < .05$, a double asterisk typically signifies alpha level $p < .01$, and triple asterisks sometimes signify alpha level $p < .001$. You may modify this scheme to fit your needs. You could, for example, use single asterisks to signify alpha level $p < .01$ and double asterisks to signify alpha level $p < .001$. (The larger probability value gets the smaller number of asterisks.) Use the same number of asterisks to denote a given alpha level in every table in the manuscript. If you need to distinguish between probability values for two kinds of statistical tests in the same table, use asterisks for one and a different symbol (e.g., daggers) for the other. Begin the first probability note on a new line at the left margin. Add subsequent probability notes on the same line.

The Body of the Table

A small set of general conventions govern how most journals format the body of a table. Follow these conventions when they enhance clarity and readability, but feel free to modify them to meet your needs, provided your modification creates a clearer, more easily understood table.

Rules

Horizontal lines, called rules, extend the full width of the table and separate the body of the table from the title and notes (Figure 5–1). Most tables contain three rules—one beneath the title, called the head rule; one above the first row of cells, called the boxhead rule; and one below the last row of cells, called the foot rule. Complex tables may include shorter horizontal lines, called spanners, which group two or more columns into a subset (see Figure 5–1).

Vertical rules rarely are used in tables and are detested by most editors because they add clutter to tables. Put vertical rules in your tables only as a last resort. Use spacing and other organizational techniques to get around the need for vertical rules. Table 5–7 shows a table with too many vertical rules. (One is usually too many.)

Eliminating vertical rules from Table 5–7 enhances the look and readability of the table, as seen in Table 5–8.

Heads and Stubs

At the top of each column of cells is a column head that identifies the content of the cells in the column (Figure 5–2). The collection of column heads is called the *boxhead*. A spanner head provides a category name for the columns under each spanner. A spanner head and the column heads arranged under the spanner head are known as *decked heads*.

	Test	Immediate Treatment			Delayed Treatment		
Head Rule > / Spanner > / Boxhead Rule >	Test	Pretest	Posttest	Diff.	Pretest	Posttest	Diff.
Spanner >				Mild Impairment			
	Listen	Data	Data	Data	Data	Data	Data
	Speak	Data	Data	Data	Data	Data	Data
	Read	Data	Data	Data	Data	Data	Data
	Write	Data	Data	Data	Data	Data	Data
Spanner >				Severe Impairment			
	Listen	Data	Data	Data	Data	Data	Data
	Speak	Data	Data	Data	Data	Data	Data
	Read	Data	Data	Data	Data	Data	Data
Foot Rule >	Write	Data	Data	Data	Data	Data	Data

Figure 5–1. Rules and spanners in a table.

Table 5–7. Percentage of U.S. Regional Population Classified as Obese

Region	Year		
	1998	**1999**	**2000**
New England	14.4	14.9	17.0
Mid Atlantic	16.7	17.8	18.4
East North Central	19.1	20.3	21.0
West North Central	18.0	19.0	19.8
South Atlantic	18.6	19.3	19.5
East South Central	20.0	21.2	23.1
West South Central	19.9	21.0	22.2
Mountain	14.1	14.5	17.1
Pacific	17.0	18.1	19.1

Note. Adapted from U.S. Public Health Service, National Center for Disease Prevention and Health Preservation. (2002). Prevalence of obesity among U.S. adults, region and state. Bethesda, MD.

Table 5–8. Percentage of U.S. Regional Population Classified as Obese

Region	Year		
	1998	1999	2000
New England	14.4	14.9	17.0
Mid Atlantic	16.7	17.8	18.4
East North Central	19.1	20.3	21.0
West North Central	18.0	19.0	19.8
South Atlantic	18.6	19.3	19.5
East South Central	20.0	21.2	23.1
West South Central	19.9	21.0	22.2
Mountain	14.1	14.5	17.1
Pacific	17.0	18.1	19.1

Note. Adapted from U.S. Public Health Service, National Center for Disease Prevention and Health Preservation. (2002). Prevalence of obesity among U.S. adults, region and state. Bethesda, MD.

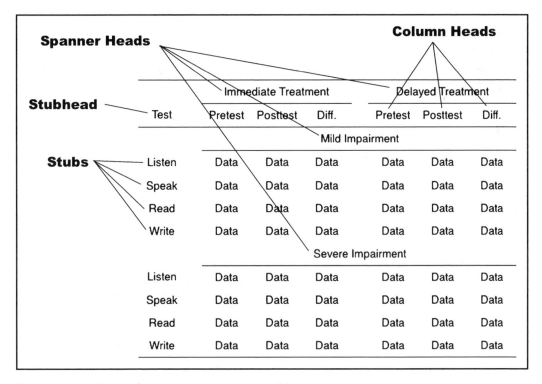

Figure 5–2. Types of heads and stubs in a table

41

The first column in a data table contains the labels for the rows. The labels for the rows are called *stubs*. The header for the column of stubs is called the *stubhead* (see Figure 5–2).

Capitalize only the first word, proper nouns, and acronyms in multiple-word heads and stubs. Nouns in heads should be singular in number unless there are multiple entries in each cell referenced by the head. The number of entries within cells, not the number of cells in a column or row, determines whether a head is singular or plural. Singular heads are much more common than plural heads. In Table 5–9, each cell in the "Region" column contains a single entry. The column takes a singular head. Each cell in the "States" column contains several entries, necessitating a plural head (see Table 5–9).

Table 5–9. Example of Single and Plural Table Heads

Region	States
Northeast	ME, MA, NY, PA
Southeast	SC, BL, AL, MS
Midwest	MI, WI, MN, IA
Northwest	WA, OR, ID
Southwest	NV, NM, AZ

Be sure that all stubheads are conceptually and syntactically homogeneous. In Table 5–10, the entries in the "Group" column on the left are not homogeneous, and the labels "Children" and "Elderly" are ambiguous. The entries in the "Age (yrs)" column in the table on the right are homogeneous (see Table 5–10).

Use descriptive labels for column heads, stubheads, and stubs. Do not force readers to refer to the text, table title, or table notes to decode vague labels such as Condition A, Condition B; Group 1, Group 2. Give them descriptive labels that can stand alone (e.g., Massed practice, Distributed practice; Treatment Group, Control Group). If you abbreviate labels to save space, ensure that the abbreviations provide enough information that readers can quickly match the abbreviations with their referents (e.g., Trt and Ctrl are more informative abbreviations for Treatment and Control than are T and C).

Arranging Rows and Columns

Arrange numeric cell entries so that comparable entries read down columns, not across rows. It is easier for readers to scan a series of numbers vertically than horizontally. That is how most of us do arithmetic calculations. In Table 5–11, comparable cell entries read across rows, not down columns, and readers must scan the

Table 5–10. Examples of Ambiguous and Nonambiguous Labels

Group	Score
Children	88
Age 20–30	96
Age 25–55	94
Elderly	97

Age (yrs)	Score
5–15	88
20–30	96
35–55	94
60–80	97

Table 5–11. Number of Migrants Leaving by State

	California	New York	Illinois	New Jersey	Pennsylvania
Rank	1	2	3	4	5
Migrants	2,170,790	1,888,936	560,003	378,495	250,958

Note. Adapted from U.S. Census Bureau. (2003). Domestic migration across regions, divisions, and states: 1995. Washington, DC.

numeric entries horizontally. The columns must be wide enough to accommodate the names of the states and seven-digit totals, which makes the table wide and shallow with excessive white space between data values. The width of this table means that if published, it will span both columns of a two-column printed page.

Rotating the table so that comparable entries read down arranges numeric entries in an easier-to-read vertical array. The columns containing numeric information are narrower, eliminating excess white space and creating a more attractive table that fits into one column of a two-column page (Table 5–12).

Arrange rows and columns to make it easy for readers quickly to see the overall point of a table. Make columns containing comparable data the same width. Arrange columns so that entries to be compared are side by side and not separated by one

Table 5–12. Number of Migrants Leaving by State

State	Rank	Migrants
California	1	2,170,790
New York	2	1,888,936
Illinois	3	560,003
New Jersey	4	378,495
Pennsylvania	5	250,958

Note. Adapted from U.S. Census Bureau. (2003). Domestic migration across regions, divisions, and states: 1995. Washington, DC.

or more columns of intervening entries. Table 5–13 shows a table in which the arrangement of rows and columns makes it difficult to compare related data elements (e.g., to see how groups compared on number of sessions and on scores in baseline, treatment, and maintenance).

Table 5–13. Number of Sessions and Overall Scores in Baseline (Bl), Treatment (Trt), and Maintenance (Mtc) Phases for Participants in Early, Middle, and Late Intervention Groups

	Session			Score		
Intervention	**Bl**	**Trt**	**Mtc**	**Bl**	**Trt**	**Mtc**
Early	12	32	8	106	128	124
Middle	10	30	6	97	106	108
Late	11	28	9	113	116	112

The same data are shown in Table 5–14, but the columns have been rearranged to place related data elements side by side. This rearrangement makes it easier for readers to compare the groups. The column heads for phases are abbreviated to minimize column width; the abbreviations are defined in the title.

Arrange rows and columns logically so that important trends and relationships are highlighted. Arrange numeric entries from largest to smallest, or vice versa, and arrange sequential events in temporal

order unless your intention in presenting the data precludes it. Table 5–15 illustrates what happens when these guidelines are not followed. The columns representing years read from right to left, contrary to the way in which we normally scan horizontal arrays. The rows are arranged vertically by region, making it difficult for readers to see how the regions rank in terms of obesity rates.

Rearranging the "Year" columns to read from left to right, and rearranging the rows in decreasing order of year 2000

Table 5–14. Number of Sessions and Overall Scores in Baseline (Bl), Treatment (Trt), and Maintenance (Mtc) Phases for Participants in Early, Middle, and Late Intervention Groups

Intervention	Early			Middle			Late		
	Bl	Trt	Mtc	Bl	Trt	Mtc	Bl	Trt	Mtc
Session	12	32	8	10	30	6	11	28	9
Score	106	128	124	97	106	108	113	116	112

Table 5–15. Percentage of U.S. Regional Population Classified as Obese

Region	Year		
	2000	1999	1998
New England	17.0	14.9	14.4
Mid Atlantic	18.4	17.8	16.7
East North Central	21.0	20.3	19.1
West North Central	19.8	19.0	18.0
South Atlantic	19.5	19.3	18.6
East South Central	23.1	21.2	20.0
West South Central	22.2	21.0	19.9
Mountain	17.1	14.5	14.1
Pacific	19.1	18.1	17.0

Note. Adapted from U.S. Public Health Service, National Center for Disease Prevention and Health Preservation. (2002). Prevalence of obesity among U.S. adults, region and state. Bethesda, MD.

obesity rates makes it easier for readers to see yearly changes in obesity rates and to see how the regions rank, as in Table 5–16.

Summary values (means, difference scores, ranges) make it easier for readers to see relationships and compare data in tables containing large blocks of numbers (Table 5–17). Column and row averages in this table highlight the differences between non-brain-injured participants and brain-injured participants and show that differences between groups are greater for reading and writing than for auditory comprehension and speech. The spanner heads (Non-brain-injured, Brain-injured) would work equally well as stubs with participant numbers indented under them. Table spanner heads often work equally well—or better—as stubs, and vice versa. Use the format that provides greater clarity and readability. (Note the large area of white space between the Participant column and the Age (yrs) column.

We could have lessened the white space by abbreviating Participant but chose not to do so because we could not devise what we considered a reasonable abbreviation.)

If a table has more than eight or ten rows, putting a blank space between every fourth or fifth row enhances readability (Table 5–18).

Aligning Heads, Stubs, and Cell Entries

Aligning heads, stubs, and cell entries can be tricky. Strive for clarity, visual symmetry, and readability. Left alignment usually works well for stubs and stubheads. Left alignment also works well for word or phrase cell entries and their column heads. Center alignment usually works well for one-word column heads and for cell entries in columns of abbreviations, acronyms, or short non-decimal numeric entries if all entries contain the same

Table 5–16. Percentage of U.S. Regional Population Classified as Obese

Region	Year 1998	1999	2000
East South Central	20.0	21.2	23.1
West South Central	19.9	21.0	22.2
East North Central	19.1	20.3	21.0
West North Central	18.0	19.0	19.8
South Atlantic	18.6	19.3	19.5
Pacific	17.0	18.1	19.1
Mid Atlantic	16.7	17.8	18.4
Mountain	14.1	14.5	17.1
New England	14.4	14.9	17.0

Note. Adapted from U.S. Public Health Service, National Center for Disease Prevention and Health Preservation. (2002). Prevalence of obesity among U.S. adults, region and state. Bethesda, MD.

Table 5–17. Participants' Ages and Scores on Tests of Auditory Comprehension (Aud), Reading (Rdg), Writing (Wrt), and Speech (Spch), Plus Their Overall Score (Z) Averaged Across the Four Tests (Means rounded to nearest whole number)

Participant	Age (yrs)	Aud	Rdg	Wrt	Spch	OA
			Non-brain-injured			
1	62	96	92	89	94	64
2	58	90	87	84	92	64
3	67	88	86	91	90	66
4	63	93	91	91	89	65
5	69	95	86	83	79	66
Mean	**64**	**92**	**88**	**88**	**89**	**63**
			Brain-injured			
1	64	74	63	59	83	69
2	66	82	71	63	87	74
3	58	67	49	32	74	56
4	62	78	62	47	63	62
5	68	61	78	75	89	80
Mean	**64**	**78**	**65**	**55**	**79**	**68**
Mean Difference	**0**	**14**	**23**	**33**	**10**	**5**

number of characters. (Some journals recommend that all stubheads and column heads be center aligned. Refer to the journal's style guide or a recent copy of the journal for guidance.)

Table 5–19 shows a portion of a table in which entries in cells are only a few characters wide. When entries in a column are only a few characters wide, center alignment usually looks better than left alignment.

Table 5–20 shows how modifying alignment of heads and cell entries can improve the appearance of a table and enhance readers' comprehension. Entries on the left are center aligned. Center alignment usually does not work well for word

or phrase entries or for numeric entries containing different numbers of digits. On the right, entries in the "State" column are left aligned, and entries in the "Out-migration" column are right aligned. Left alignment usually is best for word and phrase entries, and right alignment works well for nondecimal numeric entries.

When numeric cell entries contain decimal values, align them on the decimal points. Put a zero to the left of the decimal point for all entries containing only decimals. Carry all entries in a column to the same number of decimal places, adding trailing zeros if necessary. Put a zero ahead of the decimal point for values less than 1, but not if the value cannot be greater than 1 (e.g., proportions, correlation coefficients, significance levels). Carry all comparable values to the same number of decimal digits. Do not change the number of decimals among cells within a column.

If all entries in a column contain the same number of decimal places, right alignment and decimal alignment have the same result. If the entries in a column do not have the same number of decimal places, right alignment and decimal alignment give different results (Table 5–21).

Carrying all entries to the same number of decimal places and adding leading zeros to the left of the decimal point in pure decimal entries and aligning decimal entries on the decimal makes comparisons and mental calculations easier (Table 5–22).

Table 5–18. Net Migrations Among States, 1900–1999

Rank	State	Migration
1	Florida	1,108,514
2	Georgia	665,418
3	Arizona	577,038
4	Texas	569,957
5	North Carolina	554,268
6	Nevada	433,219
7	Colorado	402,832
8	Washington	381,552
9	Tennessee	356,907
10	Oregon	270,903
11	South Carolina	143,213
12	Idaho	136,339

Note. Adapted from U.S. Census Bureau. (2003). Domestic migration across regions, divisions, and states: 1995 to 2000. Washington, DC.

Table Width

Most journal pages are printed in two columns. Tables that fit in one column cause fewer formatting headaches than

Table 5–19. Example of Center Alignment

State	Rank
FL	1
GA	2
AZ	3
TX	4
NC	5

Table 5–20. Examples of Different Types of Alignment in Table Cells

State	Out-Migration	State	Out-Migration
California	2,170,190	California	2,170,190
New York	1,888,936	New York	1,888,936
Illinois	560,003	Illinois	560,003
New Jersey	378,495	New Jersey	378,495
Pennsylvania	250,958	Pennsylvania	250,958

Table 5–21. Examples of Different Types of Alignment for Numeric Table Entries

Right	Left	Decimal
422.35	422.35	422.35
36.7	36.7	36.7
1.38	1.38	1.38
0.444	0.444	0.444

Table 5–22. Example of Aligning Decimal Entries

Decimal
422.35
36.70
1.38
0.44

do tables spanning two columns. When you construct a table, consider its potential placement on a journal page.

Most journals do not print material in a typeface smaller than about 20 characters per inch, equivalent to an 8-pitch font in most typefaces. Single columns in most two-column journals range in width from 3 to 3¼ inches, and double-column widths range from 6½ to 7 inches. Consequently, a table cannot be more than 60 to 65 characters wide to fit into one column and not more than 130 to 140 characters wide to fit into two columns. When you estimate a table's width, count spaces as well as letters, numbers, and punctuation. Add at least three spaces for separation between columns in a table.

Tables can be placed vertically or horizontally on pages in the typed manuscript. Manuscript pages with 1-inch margins typed with a 12-point font on letter-size paper in standard (portrait) orientation average about 65 characters per line. Tables that are no more than 65 characters wide can be oriented on the page vertically (portrait page orientation). Tables that are more than 65 characters wide should be oriented on the page horizontally (landscape page orientation). Maintain consistent font size in all tables in a manuscript. Do not reduce font size to fit a wide table onto a vertically oriented page. The publisher may reduce the width of the table by printing it in a smaller font, but leave that choice to the publisher.

If a table is wider than the journal's two-column width (approximately 140 characters), it will be printed sideways on the journal page. Avoid sideways tables if you can. Sideways tables are annoying because they force readers to rotate the document to read the table, and they make it awkward for readers to alternate between the table and related text.

If a table is too tall to fit on one page, continue it on successive pages. Type Table *n* (continued) at the top of each continuation page and repeat stubheads and column heads for each section of the continued table.

Column Heads and Stubs

Keep column heads and stubs short and simple. Long heads and stubs add table width, waste space, and create clutter that gets in the way of readers' appreciation of the sense of the table. Try to keep column heads no more than a few characters wider than the widest entry in the column.

Table 5–23 shows a table in which long headings add to the width of the table and in which cell entries appear to float in an expanse of white space.

Moving words from column heads to the title reduces the width of the table but preserves its understandability (Table 5–24).

Do not repeat units of measure in a column. Put them in the column head. On the left side of Table 5–25, the percent and dollar signs in cell entries add clutter. Restricting the content of each cell to numeric information, as shown on the right side, enhances readability. We put the (%) and ($) symbols on a separate line to limit column width.

Do not include columns of values that readers can easily calculate from entries in adjacent columns. In Table 5–26, the "Difference" column adds to table width and clutter and must go.

If a column contains only a few different entries (or the same entry), eliminate the column by moving entries in it to an adjacent column or replace it with a table note. In Table 5–27, most entries in the "n" column (left) are redundant. The column should be eliminated. Moving the information to an adjacent column (center)

Table 5–23. Example of Headings That Increase Table Width

Employee Group	Number of Employees	Efficiency Coefficient	2004 Cost ($) by Division
Design	20	87	587
Finance	34	102	856
Sales	68	76	1,496

Table 5–24. Example of Headings That Do Not Increase Table Width

Group	Employees	Efficiency	Cost ($)
Design	20	87	587
Finance	34	102	856
Sales	68	76	1,496

Table 5–25. Examples of How Units of Measurement Can Be Moved to Reduce Clutter

Group	Efficiency	Cost
Design	78%	$587
Finance	68%	$856
Sales	72%	$1,496

Group	Efficiency (%)	Cost ($)
Design	78	587
Finance	64	856
Sales	72	1,496

is one option. Moving the information to a table note (right) removes clutter and makes the table easier to read.

Sometimes columns containing related information can be combined into a single column (Table 5–28), eliminating one column and lessening table width.

Use indented entries in the stub column to denote subordination, rather than adding an unnecessary column. In Table 5–29, the Conditions are subordinate elements of groups. The "Condition" column is a candidate for subordination.

Table 5–30 shows the Conditions column eliminated by subordination. Doing so creates a narrower and more readable table.

Table 5–31 shows a five-column table that is much wider than it is high, with excessive white space between cell entries.

Table 5–26. Example of an Unnecessary Column

Age	Male	Female	Difference
20–34	24	26	2
35–44	25	34	9
45–54	30	38	8
55–64	33	43	10
65–74	33	39	6

Table 5–27. Examples of How to Reduce Clutter by Removing Redundant Information

Group	n	Group (n)	Group*	Score
Young men	50	Young men (50)	Young men	96
Old men	50	Old men (50)	Old men	87
Young women	48	Young women (48)	Young women	98
Old women	50	Old women (50)	Old women	84

Note. $*n = 50$ except Young women, for which $n = 48$.

Table 5–28. Example of Combining Columns

Phase	Mean	SD	Phase	Mean (SD)
Baseline	24.8	4.32	Baseline	24.8 (4.32)
Treatment 1	29.3	4.56	Treatment 1	29.3 (4.56)
Treatment 2	36.8	3.87	Treatment 2	36.8 (3.87)
Maintenance	33.5	3.76	Maintenance	33.5 (3.76)

Subordinating "Male" and "Female" under "Income" with spanner heads eliminates redundancy and creates a better proportioned table (Table 5–32).

Converting spanner heads to stubs and subordinating "Age" to "Income" further diminishes table width and enhances readability (Table 5–33).

Table 5–29. Using Indented Entries Adds an Unnecessary Column

Group	Condition	Score
Normal	Baseline	132
	Treatment	176
	Maintenance	164
Hearing Impaired	Baseline	111
	Treatment	127
	Maintenance	118

Table 5–30. Example of Subordination

Group, Condition	Score
Normal	
Baseline	132
Treatment	176
Maintenance	164
Hearing Impaired	
Baseline	111
Treatment	127
Maintenance	118

Rounding

Rounding numeric entries in data tables often reduces column widths, although the major contribution of rounding is to increase a table's readability and make it easier for readers to see relationships and patterns in the data. Round data entries as much as you can without obscuring important relationships among data elements.

Keep the number of decimal digits under control. Round mercilessly. Do not include decimal values simply because the computer calculated them for you, or because you believe that decimal values add luster to the findings. Confine numeric entries to the number of decimal places justified by the precision of the measures used to obtain the entries. This is especially important when reporting calculated measures such as averages. Calculators and statistical software packages willingly calculate values to four or more decimal digits regardless of the precision of the measures from which the values are calculated.

Report only decimal digits that are relevant to your findings—that is, decimal

Table 5–31. Example of Excessive White Space

Age	High Income Male	High Income Female	Low Income Male	Low Income Female
20–34	40	44	38	42
35–44	46	45	47	46
45–54	52	51	54	46
55–64	44	47	50	51

Table 5–32. Example of Subordinating Elements to Improve Clarity

Age	High Income		Low Income	
	Male	Female	Male	Female
20–34	40	44	38	42
35–44	46	45	47	46
45–54	52	51	54	46
55–64	44	47	50	51

Table 5–33. Example of Converting Spanner Heads to Stubs to Reduce Table Width

Income, Age	Sex	
	Male	Female
High Income		
20–34	40	44
35–44	46	45
45–54	52	51
55–64	44	47
Low Income		
20–34	38	42
35–44	47	46
45–54	54	46
55–64	50	51

digits that co-vary with the experimental variables. Reporting too many decimal digits forces readers to read around a clutter of useless digits to get at the information they need. Report summary statistics (means, standard deviations, etc.) with two decimal digits more than are present in the observations from which the statistics are calculated.

Report correlations, proportions, and inferential statistics (t values, F values, etc.) with two decimal digits. Report percentages as whole numbers. (The first decimal digit in a percentage is equivalent to $1/1,000$, the second decimal digit is equivalent to $1/10,000$, and the third decimal digit is equivalent to $1/100,000$.) Few observations in the social and behavioral sciences merit such precision. Table 5–34 shows a table in which meaningless decimal digits compromise readability. Table 5–35 shows how eliminating trivial decimal values enhances comprehensibility; rounding to whole numbers makes it easier to see that physical activity declines during the middle years for both males and females and that a greater percentage of males than females are physically active, especially for individuals 65 years old and older.

Rounding need not and should not be confined to decimal digits. Use rounding freely to enhance readability and highlight important relationships among data elements. Pare every number in a table down to the minimum number of digits needed to convey the gist of your findings.

Ehrenberg (1977, p. 281) admonishes, " . . . round to two significant or effective digits, where 'significant' or 'effective' means digits which vary in that kind of data." He includes digits to the left of the decimal point as well as those to the right. Let's see how this might work with Table 5–36.

Table 5–36 is visually intimidating, and the point of the table is lost because of the densely packed large numbers. Table 5–37 shows how rounding simplifies Table 5–36.

In Table 5–37, cell entries are rounded to millions with a single decimal digit representing 100,000 people. The second and third decimal digits would represent 10,000 and

Table 5–34. Example Illustrating Trivial Decimal Values

Age	Male	Female
20–34	19.727	16.040
35–44	13.765	13.357
45–54	14.886	12.143
55–64	27.339	18.488
65+	38.347	22.593

Note. Adapted from U.S. Public Health Service. (2003). Percentages of physical activity including lifestyle changes among adults—United States 2000–2001. Bethesda, MD.

Table 5–35. Example Eliminating Trivial Decimal Values to Improve Clarity

Age	Male	Female
20–34	20	16
35–44	14	13
45–54	15	12
55–64	27	19
65+	38	23

Note. Adapted from U.S. Public Health Service. (2003). Percentages of physical activity including lifestyle changes among adults—United States 2000–2001. Bethesda, MD.

Table 5–36. Example of a Visually Intimidating Table

Region	Pop. 1990	Pop. 1999	Change
Northeast	50,828,313.00	51,829,962.00	−1,001,649.00
Midwest	59,869,320.00	63,242,284.00	3,372,964.00
South	85,455,793.00	96,468,455.00	11,012,622.00
West	52,837,499.00	61,150,112.00	8,312,613.00

Note. Adapted from U.S. Census Bureau. (2003). Domestic migration across regions, divisions, and stats: 1995 to 2000. Washington, DC.

Table 5–37. Example of Rounding to Improve Clarity (in Millions)

Region	1990	1999	Change
Northeast	50.8	51.8	−1.0
Midwest	59.9	63.2	3.5
South	85.5	96.5	11.0
West	52.8	61.2	8.4

Note. Adapted from U.S. Census Bureau. (2003). Domestic migration across regions, divisions, and stats: 1995 to 2000. Washington, DC.

1,000 persons, respectively, and are trivial to interpretation of the relationships conveyed in the table. (One might argue that all entries should be reduced to whole numbers.)

Table 5–38 shows another table with numeric clutter. The tens and units digits in the "Cases" column do not convey important information. The many zeros in the Hospitalization and Mortality columns also get in the way of readers' understanding of the table.

Table 5–39 shows how getting rid of meaningless decimals enhances comprehensibility.

Rescaling data-cell entries also can help rid a table of numeric clutter—for example, converting 5,000 g to 5 kg; .001 m to 1 mm; 1500 ms to 1.5 s. In Table 5–40, choosing grams as the unit of measure in the left side of the table creates numeric clutter. Rescaling the unit of measure to kilograms and rounding to one decimal

Table 5–38. Yearly Number of Cases, Hospitalization Rates, and Mortality Rates for Five Most Frequent Foodborne Pathogens

Agent	Cases	Hospitalization	Mortality
Campylobacter	102,073	0.1020	0.0010
Salmonella	75,013	0.2210	0.0078
Shigella	39,738	0.1390	0.0016
Clostridium	6,540	0.0030	0.0005

Table 5–39. Yearly Number of Cases, Hospitalization Rates, and Mortality Rates for Five Most Frequent Foodborne Pathogens

Agent	Cases (thousands)	Hospitalization (%)	Mortality (per 10,000)
Campylobacter	102	10.2	10
Salmonella	75	22.1	78
Shigella	39.7	13.9	16
Clostridium	6.5	0.3	5

Table 5–40. Example of Rescaling Numeric Values to Improve Clarity

Diet	Loss (g)	Diet	Loss (kg)
Low fat	5,378	Low fat	5.4
Low carb	8,429	Low carb	8.4
High fiber	3,294	High fiber	3.3
Standard	576	Standard	0.6

digit makes it easier for readers to see the relationships among data entries.

Empty Cells

Some cells in a data table may not contain data. The information that might appear in a cell may be trivial (e.g., cells in the diagonal of a correlation matrix representing each variable's correlation with itself). The information that might otherwise appear in a cell may be redundant (e.g., cells in the lower half of a correlation table that duplicate information from cells in the upper half, as in Table 5–41).

A column head may not apply to a cell in a particular row (e.g., Onset of disease for a healthy participant). In Table 5–42, cells to which column heads do not apply (prostate cancer in females, ovarian cancer in males) contain dashes. A cell representing cancer with very low incidence is marked with a dash and a superscript letter that refers to a table note.

Sometimes a cell does not contain data because the data were not available, could not be obtained, or were lost. Table 5–43 shows a typical way to handle such circumstances.

How should one handle blank cells? If it is obvious that a cell is empty because the cell represents information that does not exist, most journal editors recommend leaving the cell blank. If it is not obvious why a cell is blank, insert a symbol such as a dash or insert an abbreviation such as

NA for not available and explain the meaning of the symbol or abbreviation in a table note. (Center-align such symbols

Table 5–42. Example of a Table With Empty Cells

Primary Site	Male	Female
Colon	39.2	40.5
Lung	77.3	57.6
Breast	—[a]	137.1
Prostate	142.4	—
Ovary	—	16.8
Lymphatic system	22.5	19.3
Leukemia	12.9	9.6

Note. Centers for Disease Control. (2000). *United States Cancer Statistics Incidence Report.* Atlanta, GA.
[a]Fewer than 2 per 100,000.

Table 5–43. Example of How to Report Missing Data in a Table

	Session		
Participant	1	2	3
A1	47	58	63
A2	56	56	59
A3	49	—[a]	53
A4	62	60	67

Note. [a]Participant A2 did not attend Session 2.

Table 5–41. Example of Correlation Table With Redundant Values Removed

	1	2	3	4	5
1. Length	—	0.88	0.83	0.75	0.62
2. Syntax		—	0.74	0.82	0.54
3. Familiarity			—	0.93	0.64
4. Vocabulary				—	0.59

or abbreviations even though the contents of other cells in the column are aligned in other ways.) Journals differ in how they handle empty data cells, so to ensure compliance, check the publisher's style manual or the website of the journal in which your work may appear.

Reproducing Copyrighted Tables

If you wish to include a table that has appeared in a copyrighted work, you must obtain permission, usually from the publisher and from the author of the work in which the table appeared. Include a note below the table in which you give the author(s) of the work, the title of the work, the publication in which it appeared, and the copyright holder. Publishers differ in how they format such citations, but most approximate the following format:

Note. From "Effects of Sigmaphalen on Memory Impairments of Persons Diagnosed with Chronic Complaint Syndrome" by B.B. Bates and A.B. Katz, 2007. *Annals of Psychiatry, 202, 1022–1028.* Copyright 2007 by the Association for Advanced Psychiatry. Reproduced with permission of the authors and copyright holder.

A Checklist for Evaluating Tables

■ Have the data in every table been checked for accuracy?

■ Is every table necessary? Can the data from any table be presented in the text? Can tables containing related information be combined?
■ Is every table understandable without reference to information found elsewhere?
■ Are the data in tables grouped logically?
■ Is every table formatted to ensure comprehensibility?
■ Is every table referred to in the text?
■ Are all tables consistent in style and format?
■ Does every table have a brief but clear title?
■ Are table notes properly formatted and in the prescribed order?
■ Is every table sized to fit within a column or across two columns?
■ Are vertical rules eliminated?
■ Is statistical significance properly indicated?
■ Have permissions been obtained to reproduce each copyrighted table? Is credit for use given in table notes?
■ Are all tables, including titles and notes, double spaced?
■ Are unusual abbreviations and symbols defined?

References

Boone, L. (1999). *Quotable business* (p. 80). New York, NY: Random House.

Ehrenberg, A. (1977). Rudiments of numeracy. *Journal of the Royal Statistical Society. Series A (General), 140,* 277–297.

6

Constructing Data Graphs

*"Graphical excellence [is] the efficient
communication of complex quantitative ideas."*
—Edward Tufte (2001, p. 15)

Graphs are well suited for showing general relationships among data elements or for conveying a global sense of a limited set of data elements. Do not let the ease with which computer software programs transform data into graphs entice you into weighing down your manuscript with graphs to illustrate data that are better reported in the text, in a table, or not reported. Reserve data graphs for illustrating the central findings of your work.

Graph Types

If a graph is appropriate for the data, one of four basic graph types—line graph, bar graph, scatter graph, or pie graph usually will suffice. Almost all data graphs published in contemporary scientific journals are represented by these four graph types.

Line Graphs

Line graphs are useful for showing relationships between continuous variables. Continuous variables are variables that can take any value within the variable's range. Length, distance, and time are examples of continuous variables.

Line graphs can convey large amounts of information and are well suited for showing trends in data. The independent variable typically is plotted on the horizontal axis, and the dependent variable is plotted on the vertical axis. Tic marks on the axes mark coordinates for data points, as in Figure 6–1.

Data-point markers (small circles, squares, triangles) often are superimposed on data lines to provide visual anchors and make it easier for viewers to see relationships among data elements, as in Figure 6–2.

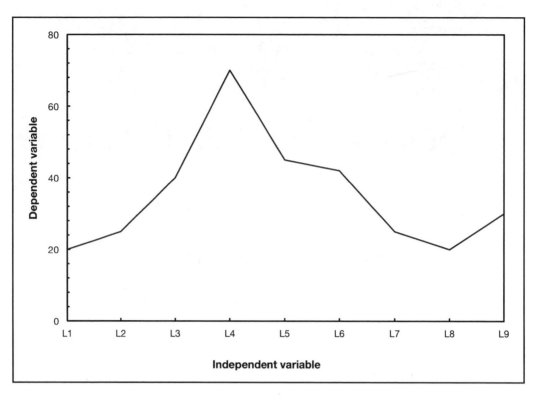

Figure 6–1. Line graph with independent variable plotted on *x*-axis and dependent variable plotted on *y*-axis.

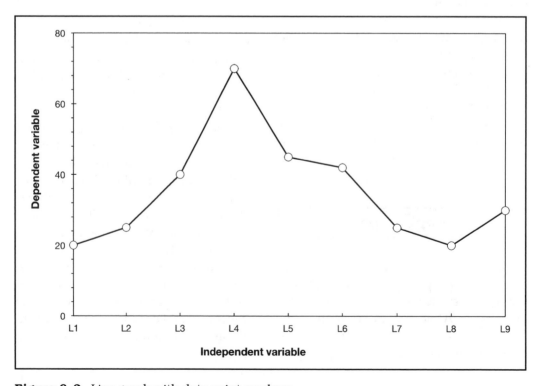

Figure 6–2. Line graph with data point markers.

Horizontal grid lines may help viewers relate data points to the scale on an axis, but too many will create visual clutter, as in Figure 6–3.

Hints for Building Effective Line Graphs

Data-Point Markers. Data-point markers give a line graph a finished look and make it easier for viewers to relate the data to the axes, so plan to include them in your line graphs. Use distinct, simple, geometric shapes (open or filled circles, squares, or triangles) for data-point markers. Make each marker about the size of the lowercase letters in the axis labels. Choose combinations of markers that retain their legibility and distinctiveness if a graph is reduced. Squares may be indistinguishable from circles when reduced in size, so avoid using combinations of squares and circles in graphs that may be reduced for publication (Figure 6–4).

Open and filled data-point markers usually tolerate reduction with little loss of visibility, so such combinations often are a good choice for graphs that may be reduced, as in Figure 6–5.

If the focus of a line graph is on the shape of a line created by many data points, all of which fall on the line, data-point markers are not needed and add clutter (Figures 6–6 and 6–7).

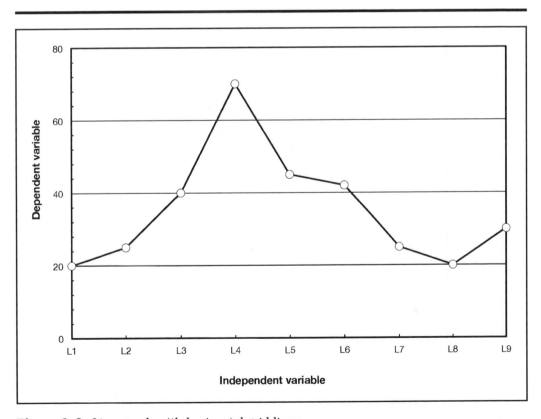

Figure 6–3. Line graph with horizontal grid lines.

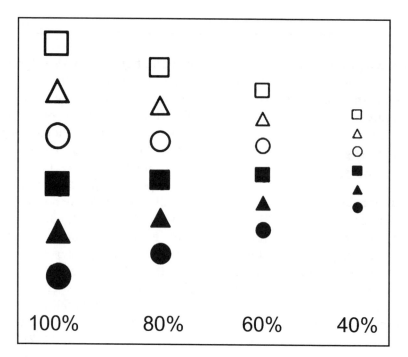

Figure 6–4. Examples of data-point markers.

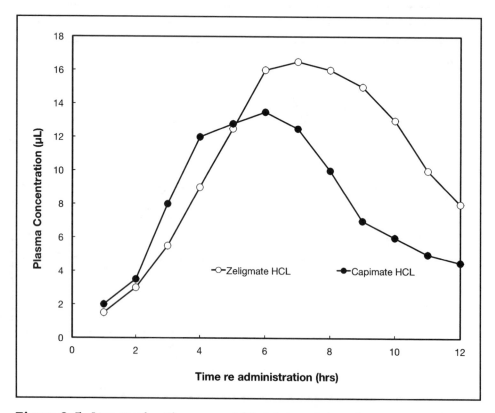

Figure 6–5. Line graph with open and filled data-point markers.

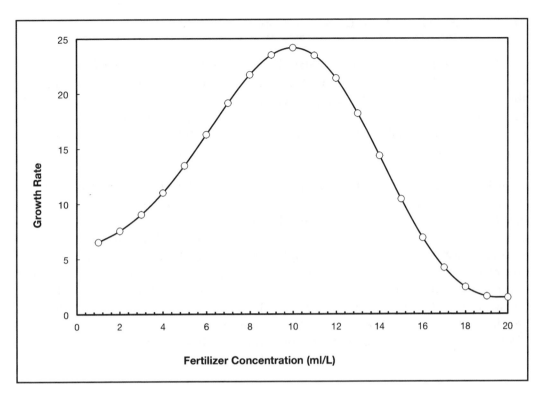

Figure 6–6. Unnecessary data-point markers in a line graph.

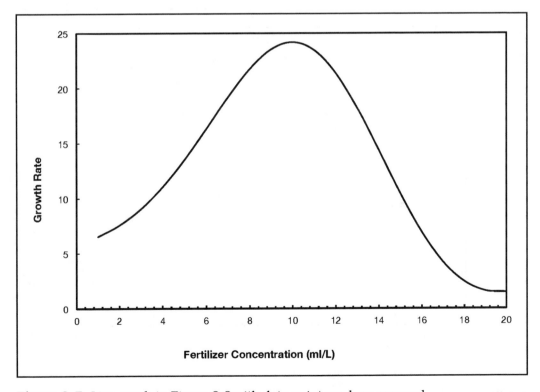

Figure 6–7. Line graph in Figure 6-6 with data-point markers removed.

61

However, if a curve is extrapolated from data points, not all of which fall on the curve, then including the data points gives viewers a sense of how well the curve fits the distribution of data points, as in Figure 6–8.

Line Styles. Different line styles also may be used to differentiate data lines in line graphs. Usually solid lines are contrasted with dashed or dotted lines. When you select line styles, choose styles with high contrast that will retain their legibility and distinctiveness when reduced. In Figure 6–9, the data lines are distinguished by different line styles. The line styles are simple and have enough contrast to tolerate moderate reduction without losing legibility. (However, we prefer to differentiate among data lines with data-markers rather than line styles. We believe that differentiating data lines with markers rather than line styles creates a cleaner, more visually appealing graph.)

Number of Data Lines. Do not try to convey too much information in a line graph. As a general principle, limit the number of data lines in a graph to five or fewer. If the data lines are separated throughout their length, viewers can tolerate more data lines, but if the data lines cross often and unpredictably, more than two may confuse viewers, and the data belong in a table, not a graph (Figure 6–10).

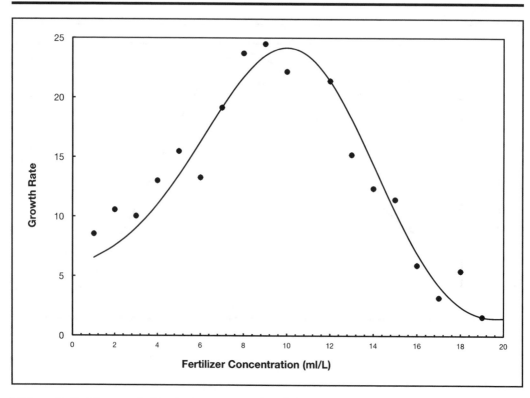

Figure 6–8. Line graph illustrating extrapolated data.

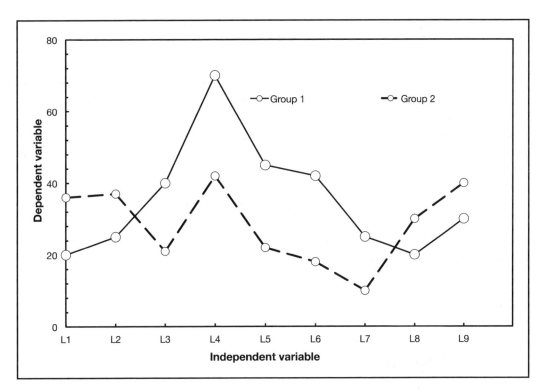

Figure 6–9. Different line styles.

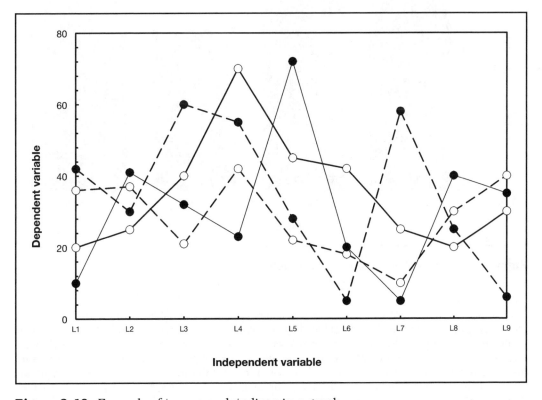

Figure 6–10. Example of too many data lines in a graph.

Bar Graphs

Bar graphs are useful for showing relationships between one or more continuous dependent variables and a categorical independent variable representing discrete components, such as the three phases of a treatment program.[1]

In vertical bar graphs (often called column graphs), the dependent variable is plotted on the vertical axis, and the independent variable is plotted on the horizontal axis. The value of each level of the independent variable is shown by the heights of the bars, as in Figure 6–11.

In horizontal bar graphs, the dependent variable is plotted on the horizontal axis, and the independent variable is plotted on the vertical axis. Horizontal bar graphs are not as common as vertical bar graphs (Figure 6–12).

Shade bars in graphs with black, gray, or patterned fill to make them stand out against the background. Proportion the

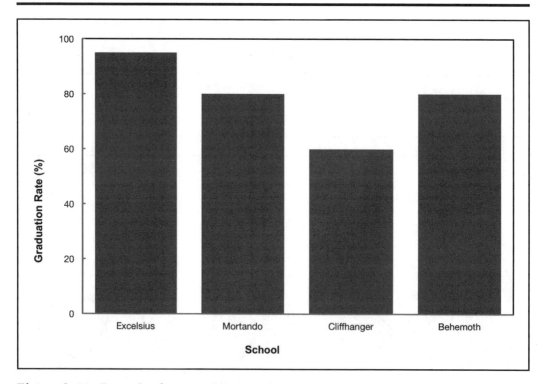

Figure 6–11. Example of a vertical bar graph.

---

[1]Categorical variables are also called discrete variables. Categorical variables are measured on a nominal or ordinal scale and include variables such as sex, species, profession, and disease. Nominal scales are not really scales. They do not order variables along a dimension but simply label them. Nominal scales classify observations into mutually exclusive groups that have no numeric value (e.g., male/female). Ordinal scales classify observations into mutually exclusive groups with an assumed rank order (e.g., poor/middle income/upper income/wealthy). The independent variables in bar graphs usually represent nominal or ordinal scales.

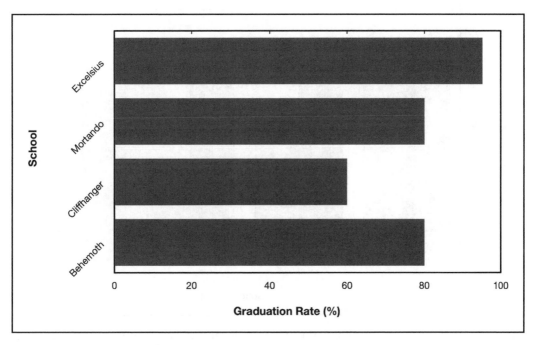

School

Excelsius

Mortando

Cliffhanger

Behemoth

0   20   40   60   80   100

Graduation Rate (%)

Figure 6–12. Example of a horizontal bar graph.

bars so that they span the data field without excessive white space. If you are using a software program such as Microsoft Excel to generate your graphs, the software will do the proportioning for you.

Do not use a bar graph to report simple data that could easily be reported in the text of the manuscript. The smaller the number of bars in a graph, the more likely it is that the data could be reported in the text. The data reported for the graduation rate bar graphs are reported more efficiently as text:

Excelsius had the highest graduation rate (97 percent); Cliffhanger the lowest (60 percent). Mortando and Behemoth had intermediate graduation rates (77 percent each).

In bar graphs showing data for more than one independent variable, the bars representing the different independent variables must be visually different. Usually this is accomplished by using shading or fill patterns within bars to identify variables and adding a legend telling how the shading or fill patterns relate to the variables. The bars within each level of an independent variable are clustered to show that they relate to the same independent variable, as in Figure 6–13.

Vertical or horizontal bar graphs with more than one independent variable can be modified so that the bar segments representing the independent variables are stacked vertically or placed one after another horizontally. Both vertical and horizontal versions are called *stacked bar graphs*. Figure 6–14 shows the percentage of daily, occasional, and former smokers and nonsmokers in the U.S population as reported in the 2002 U.S. census. We have put the largest group (nonsmokers) at the

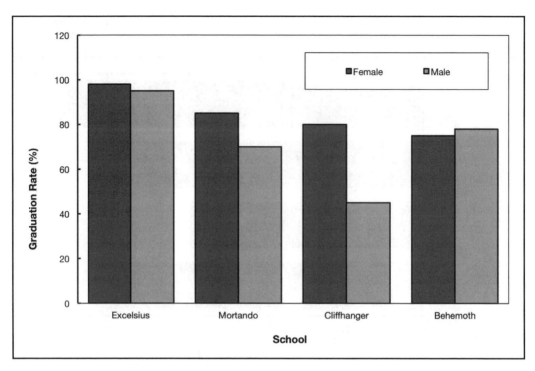

Figure 6–13. Vertical bar graph illustrating two independent variables (school and gender).

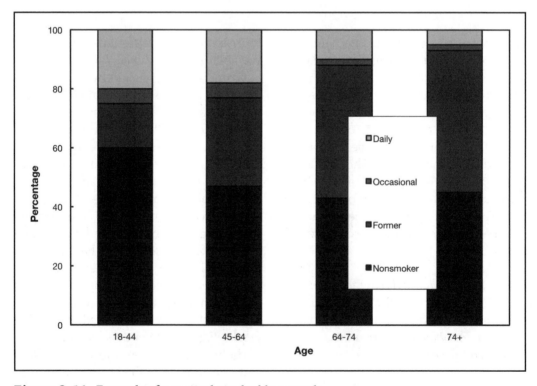

Figure 6–14. Example of a vertical stacked bar graph.

base of the bars and made lower segments darker than the segments above them, and have ordered the segments according to frequency of smoking.

Stacked bar graphs work best when the sum of the values within each bar is equal across bars, such as when bar segments represent proportions or percentages of a whole, represented by the entire bar. Stacked bar graphs make it easy to estimate the proportions represented by bar segments, but make it difficult to estimate absolute values for segments because the segments above the lowest one do not share a common baseline, as in Figure 6–15.

Hints for Building Effective Bar Graphs

When you design a bar graph, adjust the scale of the axes so that the bars span most of the data field and use space efficiently. Graphing programs will automatically generate the axes, but you may need to manually change them in order to fill the space efficiently. Use distinct fill styles to differentiate bars representing different variables. Solid fills (which actually are made up of tiny dots which yield shades of gray) almost always look better than patterned fills such as crosshatched or checkerboard patterns.

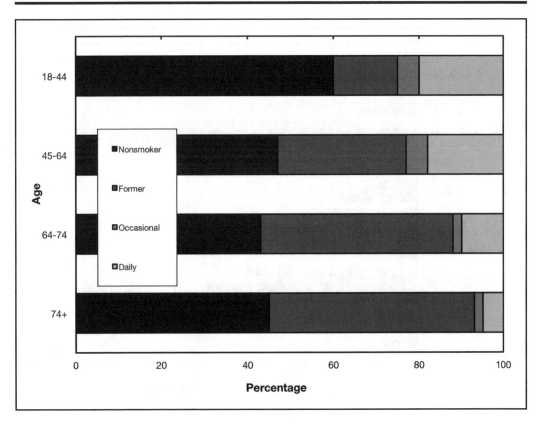

Figure 6–15. Example of a horizontal stacked bar graph.

Vertical bar graphs (column graphs) usually are better than horizontal bar graphs for conveying data in which the focus is on the absolute values of elements represented by the bars, because our eyes have an easier time comparing the height of vertical bars than comparing the length of horizontal bars. Horizontal bar graphs often are better when the labels for independent variables are too long to fit into the space available on the horizontal axis, as in the graphs shown in Figures 6–16 and 6–17.

Horizontal bar graphs also work well when the values of dependent variables move in both directions from a common reference point, such as when a variable has both positive and negative values. Placing the common reference point on the horizontal scale creates an attractive and readable graph, as in Figure 6–18.

Some combinations of bars, lines, and spaces in bar graphs may produce unpleasant visual effects (called Moirè effects) in which the visual image seems to vibrate or waver. In bar graphs, Moirè effects may appear when black or dark gray bars are separated by spaces that are roughly equal to the width of the bars or when bars contain crosshatched fill patterns, as in Figure 6–19.

Moirè effects in bar graphs can be minimized by making the bars wider than the spaces between them, butting the bars

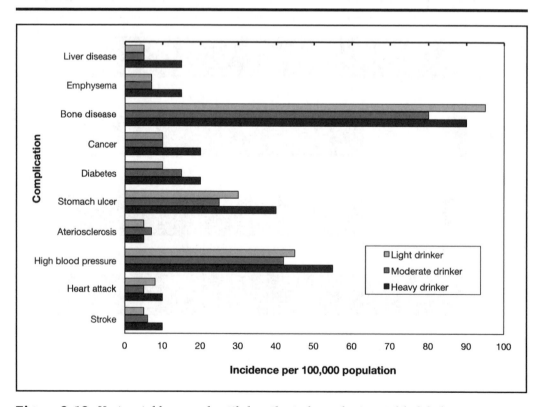

Figure 6–16. Horizontal bar graph with lengthy independent variable labels.

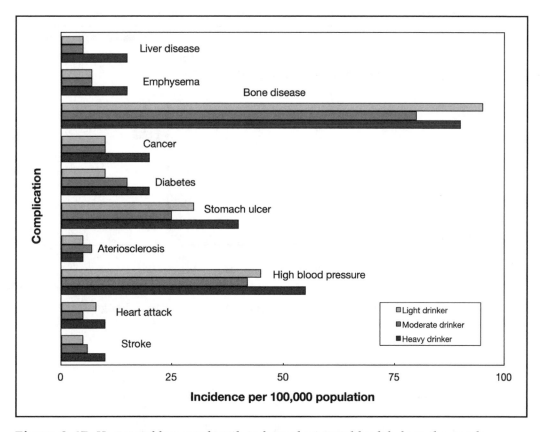

Figure 6–17. Horizontal bar graph with independent variables labels in the graph.

against each other, or using shades of gray or stippled fill patterns rather than crosshatched patterns.

Do not use more than three or four fill patterns in a bar graph or your graph will look cluttered, and viewers will have difficulty keeping the meaning of the fill patterns straight. If you need more than four fill patterns, consider making two graphs or put the data in a table.

Scatter Graphs (Scatter Plots)

Scatter graphs are useful for showing relationships between two related contin-

uous variables. The array of data points in a scatter graph shows the distribution (scatter) of observations. Clusters of data points may show interesting trends or relationships, as in Figure 6–20.

Sometimes curves representing observed or predicted trends may be superimposed on a scatter graph, as in Figure 6–21.

Hints for Building Effective Scatter Graphs

Begin the horizontal and vertical axes of scatter graphs at zero unless the range of a variable begins so far above zero as to create excessive white space, in which

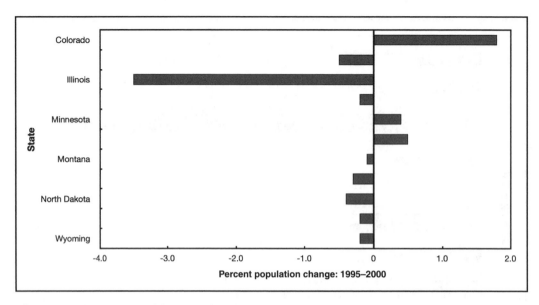

Figure 6–18. Horizontal bar graph indicating positive and negative change in the dependent variable.

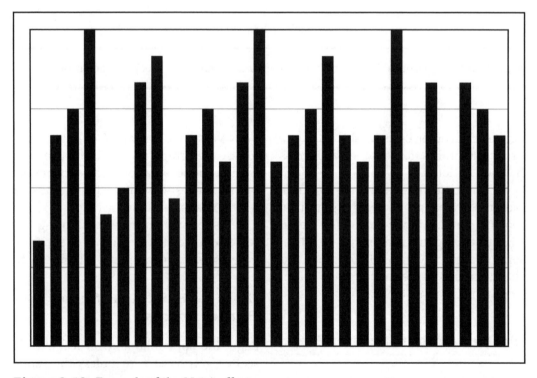

Figure 6–19. Example of the Moirè effect.

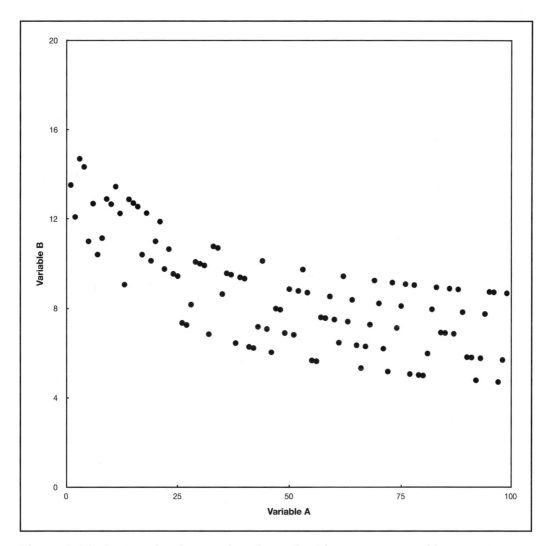

Figure 6-20. Scatter plot showing the relationships between two variables.

case you may leave out intervals between zero and the lower limit of the variable's range. Adjust the scales for the axes so that the data points span the data area. Size the symbols for data-point markers to create a visually attractive graph that will tolerate moderate reduction without loss of legibility. If you plot a curve across the array of data points, make it thick enough to be visible against the array and thick enough to tolerate reduction without loss of visibility.

Pie Graphs (Pie Charts)

Pie graphs are useful for conveying information about categorical variables

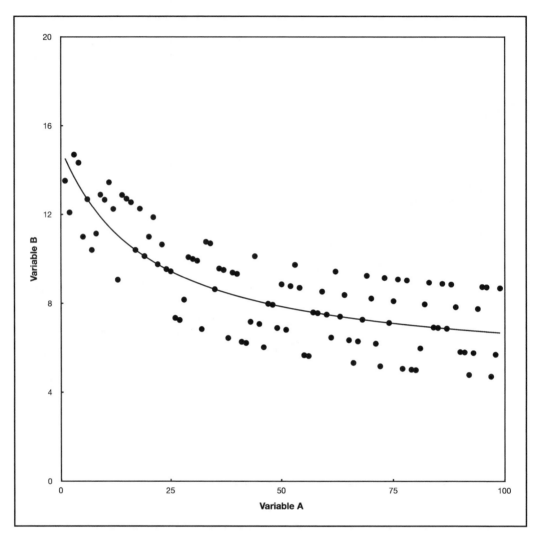

Figure 6–21. Scatter plot with trend line added.

in which the data consist of proportions or percentages. (Proportion: the magnitude of a part divided by the magnitude of the whole. Percentage: a proportion multiplied by 100.) Each segment in the pie depicts the proportion of the whole attributable to the variable represented by that segment (Figure 6–22). (Pie graphs are similar to stacked bar graphs in this respect.)

Pie segments should be distinctively shaded or filled with a distinctive pattern and labeled. Labels may include the proportion of the pie represented by each segment. Pie graphs are most practical when there are at least four or five, but no more than eight or nine segments in the graph and when the segments differ in size. (A pie graph with equal segments has no value.)

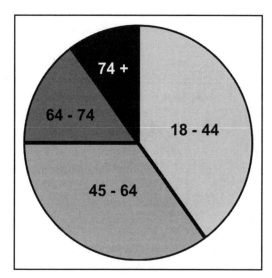

Figure 6–22. Example of a pie graph.

If a pie graph has more than eight or nine segments, the segments are likely to be so small and similar in size as to make comparisons among segments difficult or impossible (although labeling segments with their values helps). If a pie graph has more than eight or nine segments, the data usually would be better conveyed in a bar graph or a table. If the relative size of small pie segments is important, the data would be better presented in a table or in text. If a pie graph has three or fewer categories, the data usually would be better conveyed as text.

Hints for Building Effective Pie Graphs

Before you begin, check to be sure that the sum of the values representing the pie segments is equal to the total for all segments. Proportions should sum to 1 and percentages to 100. Shade segments from light to dark. Make the smallest segment the darkest segment. Arrange segments in a logical order, reading clockwise around the pie. If the segments have no inherent logical order, arrange them from largest to smallest in a clockwise direction.

Put short labels inside pie segments. (But be sure that the labels can be seen against the segments with the darkest shading.) If labels must be placed outside the pie, try to avoid the use of arrows by placing the labels adjacent to the segments they identify. Arrows almost always add to visual clutter and are almost never needed if labels are adjacent to their segments, as in Figure 6–23.

Pie graphs can be confusing to viewers, especially if the values of segments are not provided. Bar graphs usually convey the same information with less chance of confusion or misunderstanding, so choose a pie graph when the focus is on the proportions of a whole represented by levels of a variable and when precise estimation of values is not crucial. Our eyes can more accurately see differences in the lengths of bars than differences in the angles and areas of pie segments. Consequently, pie graphs are not the best way to convey information about the magnitude of values assigned to variables.

If you need several pie graphs to report related data, consider replacing the pie graphs with a stacked bar graph, which will convey the information more efficiently and make it easier for viewers to see relationships among data elements.

In research articles, pie graphs can almost always be replaced with bar graphs or tables, which provide greater precision. Pie graphs are better suited for oral presentations, in which viewers' quick grasp of general patterns and relationships is more important than the specific characteristics of the data.

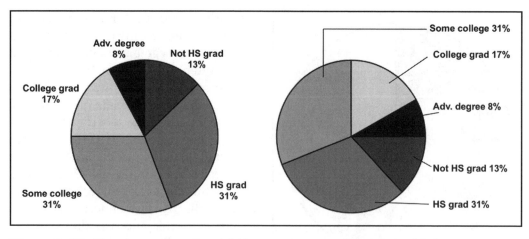

Figure 6–23. The pie graph on the right has unnecessary lines that add clutter.

Axis Titles, Scale Labels, and Legends

Most contemporary scientific publications favor a sans serif typeface such as Arial, Futura, or Helvetica for the labels, scales, and legends in graphs, even though the text is printed in a serif typeface. (Serifs are the short fine lines at the end of each major stroke in a printed letter.)

Make the typeface in axis titles slightly (one or two points) larger than the typeface in axis scales and data labels, but do not allow the difference between the largest and the smallest letters in a graph to exceed four points. Choose type sizes so that the smallest letters in a graph are no smaller than eight points after reduction. Center the title for the horizontal axis below the axis labels. The title for the vertical axis may be typed horizontally at the top of the axis (A), rotated 90 degrees and centered on the axis (B), and typed horizontally and centered on the axis (C). Do not stack letters in the title for the vertical

axis (D). Of these four options, (B) is the most common (Figure 6–24).

Type axis titles in uppercase and lowercase letters. Capitalize first words, proper names, and acronyms that require capitalization. Never print axis titles in all capital letters.

*ALL-CAPITAL MATERIAL
IS DIFFICULT TO READ
AND SEEMS TO SHOUT.*

Center the scale labels for the axes on the tic marks. Begin numerically defined axes at zero. If both axes are numeric, use a single zero to mark the beginning of both axes. If scale values include decimals, put a zero to the left of the decimal point for each purely decimal value and carry all numeric values to the same number of decimal places. Label only major increments to limit numeric clutter—leave minor scale increments unlabeled (Figure 6–25).

Putting legends outside the data field wastes space, especially if legends are placed alongside the graph. If you have

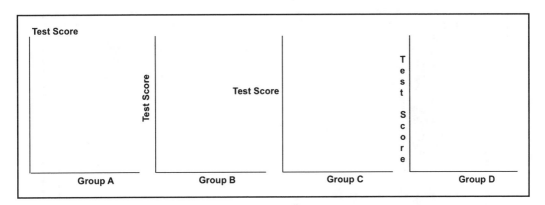

Figure 6–24. Examples of vertical axis titles.

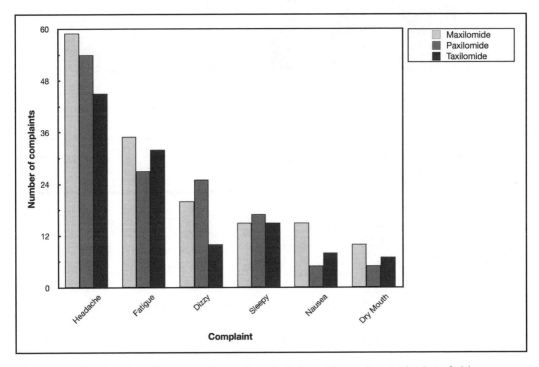

Figure 6–25. Graph with minor tic marks labeled and legend outside data field.

space, put legends inside the data field (the rectangle defined by the horizontal and vertical axes) (Figure 6–26). Sometimes labeling data elements (lines, curves, bars, data points) makes a graph easier to understand than a list of legends. If you label data elements, place the labels so that the referent for each label is clear and unambiguous. Use arrows if necessary, but only if their absence would confuse viewers.

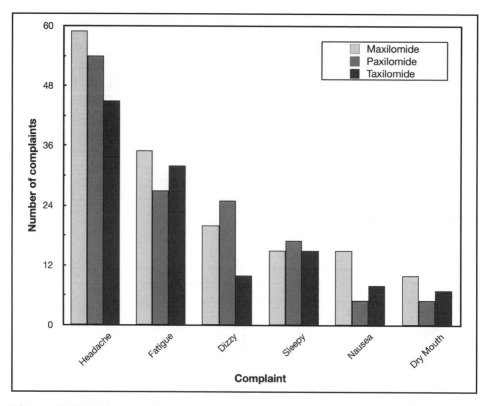

Figure 6–26. Labeling only major tic marks reduces clutter and putting the legend inside saves space.

General Principles for Constructing Data Graphs

Preparing an effective data graph requires more than plotting data points. To create an effective data graph, the creator must think, organize, and plan:

- Begin with a clear understanding of the data and what they mean.
- Decide which data are most important and most interesting.
- Select aspects of the data that address key hypotheses or research questions.
- Select data that are more effectively presented in a graph than in a table or text.

- Choose a graph format that conveys the intended message.
- Respect principles of graphic design so that the graph is clear, efficient, and effective.

A graph's appearance is almost as important as its content. Viewers should grasp the overall meaning of a data graph quickly—almost at a glance. Frills, fancy fonts, decorative flourishes, and catchy visual effects have no place in a data graph. A data graph that calls attention to its design rather than to the data it contains is a failure.

Edward Tufte (2001), a well-known advocate of simplicity in graphic design, has described what he calls the data–ink ratio. The data–ink ratio compares the amount of ink used to represent the data with the amount of ink used to make the graph. Tufte asserts that the larger the share of a graph's ink devoted to data, the better the graph. He offers four principles to guide those who build data graphs:

- Above all else, show the data.
- Maximize the data–ink ratio.
- Erase non-data ink.
- Erase redundant data ink.

Figure 6–27 is a graph that would offend Tufte.

The gridlines in Figure 6–27 add visual clutter and duplicate information provided by tic marks and scale values on the vertical axis. The fill patterns in the bars add to the clutter and carry no data information. The numbers above the bars provide the same information as the

height of the bars. (If the numbers above the bars really are important, then these data would be better presented in a table rather than a graph.)

Figure 6–28 is a cleaner version of Figure 6–27.

Line graphs almost always use less ink than bar graphs, but the amount of ink used to construct a graph should not be the primary consideration in choosing a graph type. Although line graphs tend to have more favorable data–ink/non-data–ink ratios, bar graphs sometimes do a better job of portraying important aspects of data than do line graphs, especially for categorical data.

Base your choice of graph type on the nature of the data and how the data are most accurately and effectively represented, not simply on their data–ink/non-data–ink ratios. But keep the ratio in

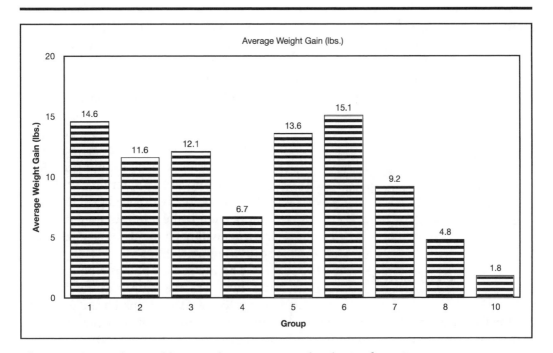

Figure 6–27. A cluttered bar graph containing redundant information.

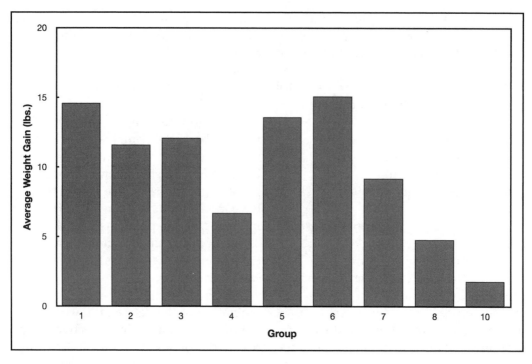

Figure 6–28. A less cluttered version of Figure 6–27.

mind as you choose a graph type and also when you build a data graph after settling on a type.

The most common sources of excessive non-data ink in data graphs are

- unnecessary grid lines,
- poorly scaled axes,
- data-related excesses (e.g., redundancy, overspecification), and
- decorative frills and flourishes.

Grid Lines

Grid marks (tics) mark intervals on axes that convey numeric information. Grid marks may extend into (usually) or away from (sometimes) the data area but should not cross the axis.

Grid lines extend tic marks across the body of the graph. Most published data graphs do not have grid lines. The purpose of a data graph is to give viewers an overall sense of data—patterns, trends, and relationships—but grid lines add visual noise that interferes with that sense. If you really do need grid lines in a graph, include the minimum number that viewers will need to relate the data to the scales (Figure 6–29).

The revised graph has a better data–ink/non-data–ink ratio, and the data are easier to see. We eliminated the gridlines and reduced the number of values on the axes by one-half (Figure 6–30).

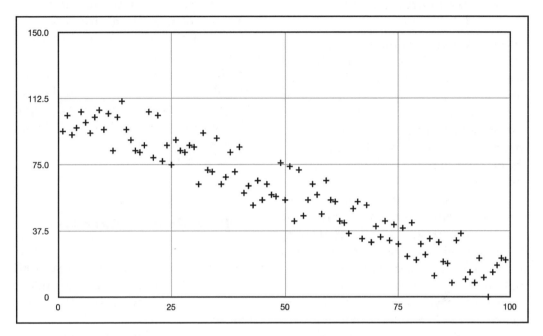

Figure 6–29. A graph with too many grid lines and axis values.

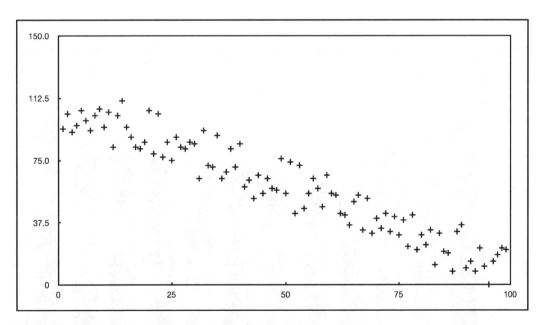

Figure 6–30. A less cluttered version of Figure 6–29.

Axes and Scales

Do not extend bars, data lines, or data points beyond either axis. End the vertical axis at the level of the highest data point or one increment beyond. End the horizontal axis one increment beyond the last bar or last data point. Size the axes so that the bars, lines, or symbols representing the data span the width and height of the graph.

Choose scale units and intervals so that the graph realistically portrays the data. Do not expand a scale to magnify differences, and do not shrink a scale to minimize them. Space values evenly and make them divisible by 10 if you can.

Do not crowd too many intervals onto an axis. Show five to ten major intervals, and space them equidistantly. Unevenly spaced intervals make it difficult for viewers to interpolate the values of data points.

Poorly scaled vertical axes are a common source of non-data ink in data graphs. Figure 6–31 shows a common source of excessive non-data ink.

If there is excessive space between the horizontal axis and the tops of the bars in a bar graph, the data lines in a line graph, or the data points in a scatter graph, break the vertical axis, delete scale values at the break (Figure 6–32).

Data-Related Excesses

Data-related excesses usually arise from overspecification of the data—redundant data markers, lines, symbols, fill patterns, and labels.

Figure 6–33 shows the percentage of U.S. adults of various ages who were reported as obese in the 2002 U.S. cen-

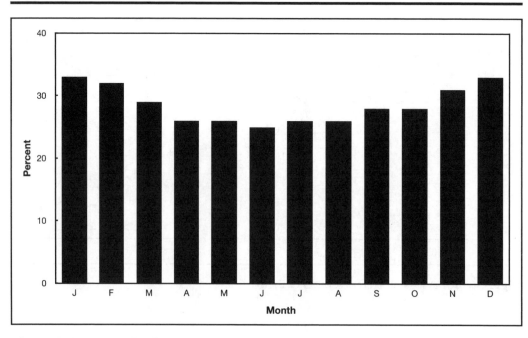

Figure 6–31. Example of a poorly scaled vertical axis.

sus. It also shows several ways in which data-related excesses creep into a data graph.

The numbers at the 5%, 15%, and 25% points on the vertical axis are not needed. Tic marks for these values suffice. The grid

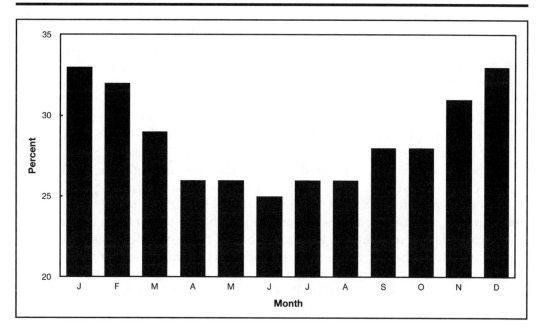

Figure 6–32. Rescaling the vertical axis in Figure 6–31 improves clarity.

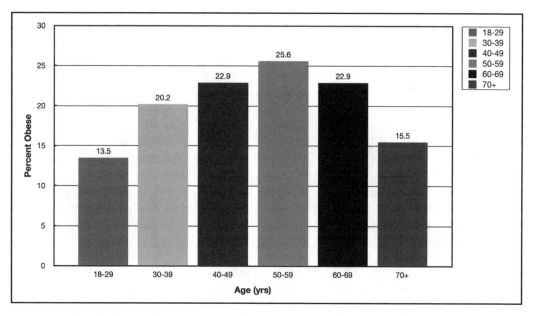

Figure 6–33. A cluttered bar graph with unnecessary redundancy of information.

lines add clutter. The legend duplicates information appearing on the horizontal axis. The bars are tagged with different fill patterns even though they represent a single variable (age). The numbers above each bar are redundant with the height of the bars.

The point of this graph is the pattern of obesity across age groups, not the percentage of obese persons in each age group. Viewers can easily estimate percentages from the heights of the bars. The pattern of bar heights effectively conveys the intended message.

Although numeric values for data points in a graph add redundancy, viewers sometimes need them, and, at least in simple graphs, the numeric values do not add much clutter. Do not routinely include them, but include them if they enhance the comprehensibility of a graph. If, however, you feel that viewers must have the

numeric values to get the point of the graph, then a table may be a better choice.

Figure 6–34 provides the same information as the preceding graph, but in a more compact, simpler, and clearer graph. Excess values have been removed from the vertical axis. Grid lines, numeric labels for bars, and the legend are gone, and a single fill pattern replaces the six fill patterns in the previous version of the graph.

Do not fragment related data by putting it into separate graphs. If you find yourself with two graphs conveying related data, combine them into a single graph.

The graphs in Figure 6–35 report the percentage of overweight U.S. male and female adults as reported in the 2002 census. Note the repetition of scales and labels in the two graphs—a sure sign that they can be combined into one.

The same data are presented in Figure 6–36 in half the space, and compari-

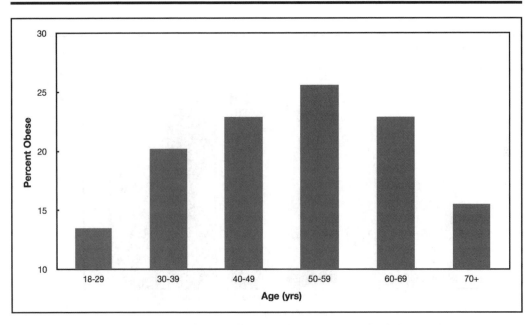

Figure 6–34. Removing grid lines, axis values, and bar shading improves clarity and reduces clutter.

sons between men and women are much easier. (We removed noninformative data points from the vertical axis and superimposed the legend on a noninformative region of the data bars to minimize graph height and width.)

Do not try to pack too much information into a bar graph. A graph in which

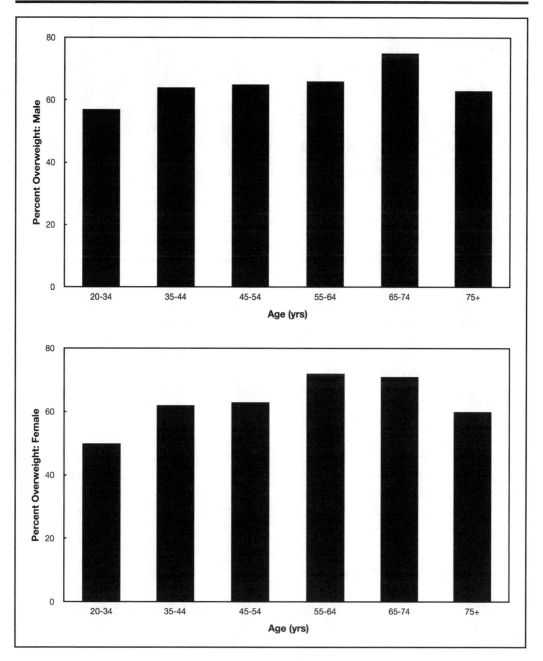

Figure 6–35. Two graphs that can be combined into one.

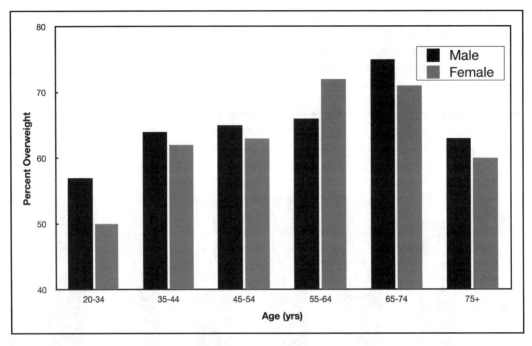

Figure 6–36. The information in Figure 6–35 combined into one graph.

data are represented by more than four or five dimensions will be difficult for most viewers to follow. If you have more than four different fill patterns in the bars of a bar graph, consider breaking the graph into two smaller graphs or put the data in a table.

Your graphs will be easier for viewers to understand if you arrange elements on axes to reflect a pattern (e.g., in chronologic order or from large to small), but be certain that the arrangement is consistent with the design of the research and with the hypotheses or questions addressed.

Decorative Frills and Flourishes

Inexpensive graphing software on personal computers provides an impressive array of choices for converting numbers into graphs. A spreadsheet program on our personal computers offers 96 graph designs, including catchy selections such as bubble graphs, donut graphs, radar graphs, cone graphs, and pyramid graphs. Although having 96 graph designs lurking within the computer is impressive, most are useless (and potentially dangerous), because it is so easy to make fancy graphs that convey little information. Many graphs in contemporary magazines, newspapers, and television seemingly emphasize decoration rather than information, usually because the graph's designer has forgotten that the purpose of a graph is clear, accurate, and efficient communication.

Submission Format

Put each graph in a manuscript destined for publication on a separate page, unless the journal specifically advises otherwise.

Every graph in an article must have a caption that provides the information readers need to get the overall point of a graph and to understand details that may not be immediately apparent from visual examination. The graph and its caption should stand alone—readers should not have to refer to surrounding text to understand the meaning of a graph. Captions are typeset separately from figures, so type your captions on a Figure Caption page. Type captions sequentially in the same font as used in the body of the manuscript. Double-space captions, and begin each caption with the word Figure and an Arabic numeral. Keep captions concise. A single sentence is best.

If you need to add explanatory material (keys to symbols, definitions, units of measurement, or explanations of features that are not immediately obvious), make the first statement a description of the data conveyed in the graph and follow with the explanatory material.

A Checklist for Constructing Graphs

Do not include a graph in a manuscript unless you can answer yes to each of the following questions:

- Is the graph necessary? Does it enhance rather than duplicate information in the text?

- Is the information in the graph complete, correct, and consistent with the text?
- Does the graph convey a single concept or conclusion?
- Is the graph clear and free of decorative flourishes and irrelevant detail?
- Are graph elements large enough and dark enough to remain legible after reduction?
- Are the scales in each graph appropriate to the data and consistent with other graphs in the manuscript?
- Is the graph consistent in style with other graphs in the manuscript?
- Are symbols or abbreviations explained in the caption or figure legend?
- Is every graph mentioned in the text?
- Are all figure captions typed sequentially on a separate page, and is each caption identified by an Arabic numeral?
- Has permission for use been obtained if the graph is reproduced or adapted from another source? Is credit given in the figure caption?

Reference

Tufte, E. (2001). *The visual display of quantitative information* (2nd ed.). Cheshire, CT: Graphics Press.

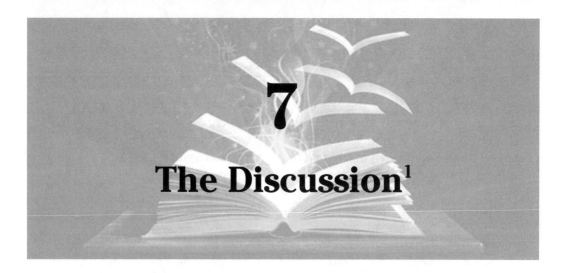

7

The Discussion[1]

"Discussion is an exchange of knowledge; argument an exchange of ignorance."
—Robert Quillen (Krarup, 1967)

The discussion puts the results in context. A well-written discussion tells readers the following:

- what the results say about the hypotheses or research questions that motivated the research;
- how new or innovative aspects of the method allow exploration of previously unknown, controversial, or inadequately understood phenomena;
- how the results relate to the findings of other investigators and to theoretical or practical issues;
- how ambiguities or inconsistencies in the results limit their interpretation or application;
- the practical applications of the results—what the results suggest about clinical or experimental methods; and
- what the results suggest about potential directions for future research.

Even for experienced writers, the discussion can be difficult to write. A well-written discussion requires that a writer

exercise judgment in separating what is important from what is not. Most studies generate far more data than should be reported, and almost all results contain inconsistencies and ambiguities that can lead a writer astray. The discussion requires that writers understand the findings and what they mean in a broad sense, beyond the confines of the research that produced the findings. A well-written discussion requires that a writer organize information to reflect its importance relative to the purposes of the research. A well-written discussion requires that a writer support assertions with data, confirm that conclusions are consistent with findings, and ensure that speculations and hunches are clearly labeled.

How to Begin the Discussion Section

Findings-Based Openings

Unlike the introduction, which progresses from general to specific, the discussion progresses from specific (the findings) to

[1]Unless otherwise noted, the examples in this chapter, and the citations within them, are fictitious.

87

general (what the findings mean). Discussions in most contemporary research articles begin with a summary of major findings—those that directly relate to the hypotheses or research questions.

> *The results of this study show that failure to perceive a target during one panoramic search trial does not reliably predict failure to perceive that target on subsequent trials. Our participants were no more likely to miss a previously missed target than to miss a previously perceived target. In fact, the probability of target perception was slightly but not significantly higher for previously missed targets than for previously perceived targets.*

Findings-based openings often begin with a lead-in phrase, such as

> *The results of this (the present) study suggest . . .*
>
> *The results of this investigation confirm . . .*
>
> *Our results show . . .*

Summaries of major findings usually consist of a series of assertions about the findings and a recapitulation of the evidence supporting each assertion.

> *The results of this study [lead-in] show that norms for the Social Adaptability Scale (SAS) are not valid indicators of social adaptability for poorly educated adults [assertion]. Education accounted*

> *for almost one-third (31%) of the variance in SAS scores. Education had a much stronger effect than either age, which accounted for less than 7% of the variance, or ethnicity, which accounted for less than 5% of the variance [evidence].*

> *Our results suggest that [lead-in] paracriptine therapy does not improve normal elderly adults' mental flexibility [assertion]. Changes on tests of mental flexibility were no greater for participants taking the recommended regimen of paracriptine than for participants receiving a placebo [evidence].*

Although boilerplate[2] lead-in phrases such as "the results of this study show" are common, they are by no means necessary, and they usually add unnecessary words. Dispensing with the lead-in aids precision and enhances readability.

> *The norms for the Social Adaptability Scale (SAS) are not valid indicators of social adaptability for poorly educated adults [assertion]. Education had a much stronger effect than either age . . . [evidence]*

> *Paracriptine therapy does not improve normal elderly adults' mental flexibility [assertion]. Changes on tests of mental flexibility were no greater . . . [evidence]*

Findings-based openings have several advantages. Beginning the discussion

---

[2]*Boilerplate* is text that is used multiple times without changes. *Boilerplate* originally referred to standard-size steel plates manufactured for steam boilers. In the early 1900s, *boilerplate* referred to type that was stamped or cast in metal and distributed to newspapers to be printed verbatim. *Boilerplate* also refers to standard provisions in contracts and other legal documents.

with major findings links the hypotheses or research questions to the results and contributes to coherence. Because it is such a common organizational device, readers expect to see major findings summarized and related to hypotheses or research questions at the beginning of the discussion. Readers who skim an article will look at the first few paragraphs in the discussion for enumeration and discussion of the most important findings and are likely to miss them if they are placed later in the discussion.

Purpose-Based Openings

Sometimes the discussion begins by restating the purpose of the research, the hypotheses, or the research questions.

We evaluated three hypotheses concerning the effects of brain-injury on adults' proverb interpretations: (1) that proverb familiarity and proverb abstractness would affect both groups' performance; (2) that brain-injured adults' performance would be inferior to that of non-brain-injured adults; and (3) that abstractness would have disproportionately large effects on brain-injured adults' performance. The results supported all three hypotheses . . .

This study was designed to determine if adults with right-hemisphere brain injuries differ from adults with left-hemisphere brain injuries when they are asked to judge the plausibility of noncontextual transitive active sentences. The results suggest that they do, but that severity of brain injury has potent effects on the differences obtained . . .

Some style guides assert that writers should not begin the discussion by restating purpose, hypotheses, or research questions. Nevertheless, purpose-based openings sometimes have merit. If the results section ends with incidental findings related only tangentially to the purpose, hypotheses, or research questions, a purpose-based opening may help readers get back to the point of the research. Purpose-based openings are best suited for situations in which readers are likely to have strayed from the point of the research or need some easy reading after struggling through complex results.

Purpose-based openings have several disadvantages. They may add unnecessary words by restating material that readers already know. They may disrupt the natural flow of information from the results to interpretation of the results. They may tempt the writer to spend more words describing the purpose than readers need. If you choose a purpose-based opening, keep it short, simple, and direct. You gave your purpose, hypotheses, or research questions in the introduction. Readers need only a reminder, not a complete restatement of the earlier material. Focus the discussion on what the results say about your hypotheses or research questions, not on the hypotheses or questions themselves.

Procedures-Based Openings

A few research articles begin the discussion by mentioning important aspects of procedures before moving on to major results.

We measured five aspects of story grammar in stories written by third-grade children, representing children with normal language development, children with language delay greater than 6 months, and children with attention-distractibility syndrome [procedures]. Three of the five story grammar measures reliably separated the three groups . . . [results]

A single-subject, multiple-baseline, crossover design with baseline, treatment, and maintenance phases was used to evaluate the efficacy of emotive therapy in alleviating depressive symptoms in seven clinically depressed adults [procedures]. Emotive therapy strongly reduced depressive symptoms in all seven, but five of the seven failed to maintain reduced symptom levels during maintenance . . . [results]

Procedures-based openings are not common in contemporary research articles. They have several faults. They move the focus away from interpretation of results. They usually add unnecessary words. They disrupt the natural flow of information from the results to interpretation of the results. Use procedures-based openings sparingly. Reserve them for situations in which the procedures are unusual or innovative, strongly affect your interpretation of the results, or both.

How to Organize the Discussion

Because discussion sections have a propensity toward wanderlust, tell yourself, "Get to the point," as you begin writing the discussion—the "point" being, what do the results mean beyond the context of this particular work? (the "so what?"

question). The most effective way to begin the discussion is with a strong assertion about the major findings.

Paracriptine therapy does not improve normal elderly adults' mental flexibility.

Then back up your assertions with the results that support them.

End-of-treatment changes in Minnesota Mental Flexibility Test (MMFT) scores of participants who received paracriptine therapy were not significantly different from the MMFT scores of participants who received a placebo. Neither the paracriptine group nor the placebo group experienced a significant change in MMFT scores between the beginning and end of treatment. Subjective ratings of mental flexibility by participants and their spouses did not change from the beginning to the end of treatment for either group.

Relate your major findings to relevant findings from other work, to significant theoretical or practical issues, or both.

We believe our findings to be a better indicator of paracriptine's effects on mental flexibility of normal elderly adults than are the findings of Blackstone (2003) and Hogue (2004). Blackstone used a single-blind design in which participants did not know if they received paracriptine or a placebo, but those who measured participants' mental flexibility knew which participants were receiving paracriptine and which were receiving the placebo. Our study used a double-blind design in which neither the participants nor those who tested them knew who was receiving paracriptine and who was receiving the placebo. It is well known that double-blind designs are superior to single-blind designs in minimizing the potential effects of investigator expectations on the results obtained.

Participants in Hogue's study were residents of extended-care facilities. Hogue did not screen participants for the presence of depression—an important oversight because it is well known that the incidence of depression is higher in residents of extended-care facilities than in the normal population (Danver & Villamonte, 2000) and because it also is well known that depression negatively affects cognition, including, presumably, mental flexibility (Mazzolo, Friederich, & Lyon, 2002).

As a practical matter, our results suggest that paracriptine does not improve normal elderly adults' mental flexibility and should not be prescribed for that purpose.

If there are less important but relevant findings in the results section, discuss them after you have discussed the major findings, but be sure to limit the discussion to issues directly related to the topic of the research or to interpretation of the findings. Discuss only findings that are clearly supported by the data, consistent with the design of the study, and related to issues identified in the introduction. Do not introduce new findings in the discussion, and do not take readers down tangential byways that are interesting to you but which do not have direct ties to the results.

Discussion sections of most manuscripts under editorial review are too long. Usually they are too long because writers pull in incidental findings that have little to do with the purpose of the research or engage in speculation not supported by the data. Your objective in the discussion is to offer and support the most plausible interpretation of the findings, based on the evidence provided by the data. The discussion is not the place for idle speculation, wild hunches, or irrelevant comments.

If your findings have limitations, discuss them.

Our findings do not address paracriptine's potential therapeutic effects on depression. None of our participants reported symptoms of depression, and none had been diagnosed as depressed in the 10 years prior to entry into our study.

If your findings logically support a reinterpretation of your hypotheses or research questions or if they offer an alternative explanation for previous findings, discuss them.

Our findings suggest that improvements in mental flexibility reported by Blackstone (2003) and Hogue (2004) may, in fact, represent paracriptine's effect on depression.

If your findings suggest that additional research is needed, tell readers why the research is needed and what specific issues or problems the research should address. Do not simply say that additional research is needed and leave it at that.

Clearly, additional study of the effects of paracriptine on depression and cognition is warranted. We found no meaningful effects of paracriptine on the mental flexibility of normal elderly adults—findings that conflict with those of Blackstone (2003) and Hogue (2004). On the other hand, several studies have shown positive effects of paracriptine on chronic depression. We do not know if Blackstone and Hogue's findings represent lessened depression or specific improvement in cognitive function. Additional work might profitably focus on determining if paracriptine's purported efficacy for improving mental flexibility actually represents efficacy in lessening depression. Such work would also be useful in further explaining relationships between depression and specific characteristics of cognitive functions.

The discussion should be complete in itself. Readers should not have to look back at preceding sections to understand what is said in the discussion. But do not repeat material from a preceding section word-for-word in the discussion.

How and When to Use Headings to Enhance Readability

Headings help readers see the organization of the discussion. Generally, longer discussions need more headings. Shorter discussions (10 to 12 paragraphs or fewer) may not need any headings and are unlikely to need more than two or three. As a discussion gets longer, the usefulness of headings increases.

We looked at the discussion sections in 70 research articles recently published in behavioral science and medical journals to get a sense of discussion lengths and the relation between the length of the discussions and number of headings provided. The 70 discussions ranged in length from 1 paragraph to 28 paragraphs (average length = 11 paragraphs). Most (34%) were seven, eight, or nine paragraphs long. Less than 20% were more than 14 paragraphs long, and less than 10% were less than five paragraphs long. The Pearson correlation between discussion length and number of headings was $r = .72$ ($p < .01$), suggesting a moderately strong relationship between the two. Ninety percent of discussions with 10 or fewer paragraphs had no headings, and none had more than two headings. Seventy-six percent of discussions with more than 10 paragraphs had headings, averaging about one heading for every five paragraphs.

Although there was great variety in the lexical content of headings that reflected differences in content among the discussion sections, a few headings occurred fairly often:

- Major Findings,
- Implications (Clinical Implications),
- Directions for Future Research, and
- Summary/Conclusions.

Use headings to help organize a discussion and to help readers comprehend it. If the discussion addresses several topics and if topics get several paragraphs each, headings likely will be needed to guide readers from topic to topic. Use headings to mark changes in topic, but do not sprinkle the discussion with headings simply to increase white space. You may need a heading for every five or six paragraphs, depending on where changes in topic occur.

Combined Results and Discussion Sections

Some journals permit combined results and discussion sections. Sometimes a combined results–discussion section is more readable than separate sections. If results are complex and address several research questions, readers of a continuous string of results related to several questions are likely to lose their way. Discussing each set of results before moving on to present the next set will help them stay on track.

Combined results and discussion sections may be organized in either modular or topical fashion. In modular organization, all the results are presented at once and the discussion follows. Modular organization is equivalent in format to separate results and discussion sections, but with one heading instead of two. Modular format has the same advantages and disadvantages as separate sections, although it saves a bit of space by eliminating one heading. Modular organization of combined results and discussion usually is harder for readers to follow than separate sections, so it makes little sense to choose this format for the combined section.

A better organizational choice for combining results and discussion is topical organization. In topical organization, discussion follows each result. Topical organization is easier for readers to follow than modular organization, especially when results and statistical analyses are complex.

No global rules govern writers' choice of separate or combined results and discussion, although individual journals may require one or the other. If you have a choice, choose the option that portrays your findings and their meaning in the clearest, most efficient, and easiest-to-read format.

How to Close the Discussion

Confine the discussion to issues that relate to important theoretical or practical concern. Do not comment on incidental details of the results. Be especially careful not to make unsupported claims about your results—a common fault in manuscripts under review. If inferences or implications are justified, include them but do not go beyond the limits of the data. Clearly identify speculations and be certain that the speculations are unequivocally supported by the results.

The last paragraph or two in the discussion should provide readers with a take-away message that you want them to remember. The take-away message may tell

- why the findings are important;
- how the findings relate to larger practical or theoretical issues;
- what theoretical positions or practical assumptions are supported or challenged by the findings;
- how new and innovative aspects of the method explain previously unknown, controversial, or inadequately understood phenomena; and
- the practical applications of the findings—what the findings suggest regarding clinical or experimental methods.

End the discussion on a positive note. Do not qualify the results to death. Do not equivocate or apologize. End the discussion with what is important and noteworthy about your findings. Do not close the discussion by discussing the limitations of your work, describing incidental findings, or engaging in empty conjecture. A closing sentence or two about potential directions for continued research may be appropriate, but only if they arise naturally.

Conclusions

Some journals permit a final conclusions section in which major conclusions are briefly enumerated. Conclusions sections usually are one paragraph long, rarely contain more than three paragraphs, and almost never contain headings.

Conclusions
Paracriptine had neither significant nor clinically meaningful effects on normal elderly adults' mental flexibility. Participants receiving the recommended regimen of paracriptine showed no greater changes on a test of mental flexibility than participants receiving a placebo in our double-blind study. Our results do not support previous reports of paracriptine's positive effects on mental flexibility (Blackstone, 2003; Hogue, 2004). We suggest that these previously reported positive effects may reflect paracriptine's effect on depression rather than mental flexibility.

Hedging Language

Hedging language—language with which writers qualify interpretations and con-clusions—is common in discussion sections of research articles.

Beck and Bond apparently were not aware of Cutter, Cooley, and Camelback's previous work.

These data suggest that 12 hours of video gaming per day has potentially irreversible negative effects on familial harmony.

It appears unlikely that differences of this magnitude could have occurred by chance.

Writers hedge with verbs (seem, tend, appear, indicate, suggest), auxiliary verbs (may, might, could), adverbs (often, usually, sometimes), adjectives (probable, likely, possible), or lead-in clauses (It could be . . . , It seems likely . . . , It would appear). Hedging language is conventional in much academic writing, conveying respect for others' work and permitting a writer to back off from claims of absolute truth. There is nothing wrong with hedging language, provided it is not used to excess and provided it does not lead to awkwardness. But look carefully at lead-in hedges, such as, *It seems likely that . . .* or *It appears that . . .* Such lead-ins usually add extra words. If you have to begin a sentence with a hedge, try for a single word rather than a phrase:

- *Seemingly* for *It seems likely that . . .*,
- *Apparently* for *It appears that . . .*, or
- *Perhaps* for *It may be that . . .*

The next two chapters address the Title and Abstract, which are easier to write after completing the introduction, method, results, and discussion sections of your manuscript.

Guidelines for Writing the Discussion

- Emphasize what is important about the findings.
- Prefer findings-based openings.
- Arrange findings in decreasing order of importance.
- Discuss more important findings in greater detail than less important findings.
- Address the practical or theoretical importance of the findings.
- Do not engage in speculation not supported by the findings.
- Keep the discussion lean, simple, and direct.
- Prune your hedges.

Reference

Krarup, A. (1967). *The school day begins: A guide to opening exercises, grades kindergarten–12* (p. 200). New York, NY: Hobbs, Dorman & Co.

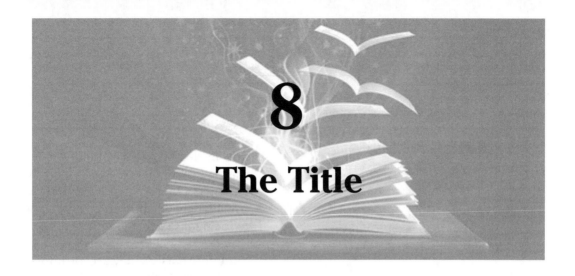

8

The Title

"Empty heads are very fond of long titles."
—German Proverb

The title of a scientific paper concisely defines the topic and scope of the paper. A well-written title in a few words expresses the topic of an article and provides key information to readers who may be searching indexes or lists of titles for papers related to a topic. A well-written title tells the reader enough about the purpose and content of a paper to permit an informed decision about whether or not to read the paper. A well-written title is clear but concise, and devoid of redundancy, useless words, and irrelevant detail. Titles need not be complete sentences but should be syntactically well formed. Most are phrases composed of key words (usually nouns and adjectives) linked by a few connecting words (conjunctions, prepositions, and sometimes articles), as in these examples.

Cervical dystonia as first manifestation of multiple sclerosis (Rüegg, Bühlmann, Renaud, Steck, Kappos, & Fuhr, 2004)

Stimulus processing constraints in audition (Dyson & Quinlan, 2004)

Word frequency and lateralization of lexical processes (Coney, 2005)

The key words in titles identify independent variables, dependent variables, methodology, or participants, as in the following examples, wherein key words are in italics.

Effects of *frequency* and *predictability* on *eye fixations* in *reading* (Rayner, Ashby, Pollatsek, & Reichle, 2004)

Orthographic neighborhood and *concreteness* effects in a *lexical decision* task (Samson & Pillon, 2004)

Awareness of limitations, goal setting, and *rehabilitation outcome* in patients with *brain injuries* (Fischer, Siegfried, & Trexler, 2004)

Title Format

Indicative Titles

Titles of contemporary scientific papers take several forms. Most are indicative. An indicative title simply identifies the topic of a paper.

Role of stimulus-driven and goal-driven control in saccadic visual selection (vanZoest, Donk, & Theeuwes, 2004)

Carotid artery stenting with routine cerebral protection in high-risk patients (Lin et al., 2004)

Effects of speech and print feedback on spelling by children with autism (Schlosser & Blischak, 2004)

Informative Titles

Informative titles convey both a topic and a major conclusion. Such titles typically contain verbs such as prevent, predict, cause, effect, and the like.

Cognitive and SPECT characteristics predict progression of Parkinson's disease (Dujardin et al., 2004)

Directional control of reaching is preserved following mild to moderate stroke (Reinkensmeier, Cole, Kahn, & Kamper, 2002)

Knowledge about the probability of change affects change detection performance (Beck, Angelone, & Levin, 2004)

Beta-blockers prevent cardiac events in Japanese patients with myocardial infarction (Ishikawa et al., 2004)

Not everyone is beguiled by informative titles. Rosner (1990) asserts that informative titles (which he called assertive sentence titles)

■ contain unnecessary words (usually verbs);
■ have a dogmatic ring, because the title becomes an assertion;

■ are written in the present tense, although results traditionally are written in past tense;
■ may mislead readers by boldly stating results that are stated more tentatively in the paper itself; and
■ trivialize the scientific report by reducing it to a one-liner.

Many journals do not accept informative titles, primarily because informative titles too often violate the principle of external validity—the extent to which the results of an experiment can be generalized to a population from which a sample is drawn. Unequivocal generalization of the findings of an experiment from a study group to a population is almost never possible because participant selection, study design, measurement procedures, controls, and data analysis methods limit generalization of the results from a sample to a population. The next assertive sentence title (from a 1986 study of respiratory infections in elderly adults) shows how this can happen.

Oral hygiene reduces respiratory infections in elderly bed-bound nursing home patients (Takeyoshi et al., 1996)

This title asserts that oral hygiene reduces respiratory infections in elderly bed-bound nursing-home patients. The abstract, however, suggests that the results were less conclusive (emphasis added by us):

During oral care for six months, *febrile days did not improve*, but degradation of febrile days were prevented by oral care for a *limited number* of patients. We suggest that oral care may be useful to some extent in elderly patients to prevent respiratory infections.

The problem here is not that the title was an informative one, but that it did not provide a true picture of the results. Adding qualifiers to the title makes it less misleading but diminishes its force:

Oral hygiene continued for 6 months may reduce respiratory infections in some elderly bed-bound nursing home patients

Informative titles for research articles in the behavioral sciences and medicine are rare. We collected a sample of 300 titles of articles from the Medline database maintained by the National Library of Medicine. The titles represented articles in psychology, neuroscience, language, and medicine. We found fewer than a dozen informative titles in the 300. About half were titles for nonresearch articles published in newsletters or general-interest publications.

Antibiotics fail to prevent heart attacks (Harvard Health Publications, 2004)

Statins prevent first strokes . . . and they may improve the chances of recovery after a stroke (Schwamm, 2004)

If a research article had an informative title, it usually was a study with animal subjects or an experiment with cell cultures, bacteria, and the like, as in the following examples.

Early administration of nicotinamide prevents learning and memory impairment in mice induced by 1-methyl-4-phenyl-1, 2, 3,

6-tetrahydrpyridine (Yang, He, Wang, & Adams, 2004)

Asialoerythropoietin is not effective in the R6/2 line of Huntington's disease mice (Gil, Leist, Popovic, Brundin, & Petersen, 2004)

Heat shock protein 70(HSP70) does not prevent the inhibition of cell growth in DU-145 cells treated with TGF-beta1 (Ogawa et al., 2001)

The rarity of informative titles in medicine and the behavioral sciences suggests that journal editors in those disciplines do not encourage them. Editors of biomedical and biochemical journals seem more permissive, perhaps because the effects of confounding variables may be better controlled and generalization of results better supported in the biological sciences, even though the validity of the generalizations cannot be fully established.

An informative title on a research article is almost certain not to satisfy requirements for external validity. Unless your work is headed for a journal that favors informative titles, use them with caution.

Question Titles

Some authors write titles as questions, as in these examples:

Does delirium increase hospital stay? (McCusker, Cole, Dendukuri, & Bbelzile, 2003)

Does donor cause of death affect the outcome of lung transplantation? (Ciccone et al., 2002)

Can we prevent aspiration pneumonia in the nursing home? (Oh, 2004)

Do patients with Parkinson's disease benefit from embryonic dopamine-cell transplantation? (Freed et al., 2003)

Question titles, like informative titles, have weaknesses. Such titles may pique readers' interest, but they are less efficient than indicative titles because they contain unnecessary words (verbs such as do, does, can, is, and will). More importantly, question titles may cause indexing and abstracting systems to generate weird or unintelligible results because the systems are not designed to separate unnecessary words from important words. Question titles also may seem condescending to readers and trivialize the work to which they are attached because they have only three possible answers—yes, no, or maybe.

Titles can, of course, be written as open-ended questions that cannot be answered with yes, no, or maybe. Open-ended question titles yield less trivial titles, but add extra words:

To what extent does delirium affect length of hospital stay?

What are the relationships between cause of death and the outcome of lung transplantation?

How can we prevent aspiration pneumonia in the nursing home?

Open-ended question titles, like yes–no question titles, may lead indexing and abstracting systems astray. Rewriting question titles as indicative titles increases clarity and promotes accurate indexing:

Delirium and length of hospital stay

Donor cause of death and outcome of lung transplantation

Preventing aspiration pneumonia in nursing homes

Use questions as titles for research articles cautiously. Question titles seem more appropriate for newsletters, tutorials, or oral presentations, where they help capture readers' or listeners' interest, than for research articles, where the readers' interest in the topic can be presumed.

Indicative titles are far more common than either assertive sentence titles or question titles in contemporary scientific publications. Of the 300 titles we extracted from Medline, 280 (93%) were indicative titles. Twelve (4%) were informative (assertive sentence) titles. Eight (3%) were question titles.

Hanging Titles

Hanging titles have two parts—a main title and a subtitle separated from the main title by a colon. Most hanging titles are made up of an indicative main title and an indicative subtitle. The main title identifies the topic, and the subtitle gives additional information:

Rate and loudness manipulation in dysarthria: Acoustic and perceptual findings (Tjaden, & Wilding, 2004)

Albumin-bound polyacrolein: Implications for Alzheimer's disease (Siedler & Yeargans, 2004)

Some hanging titles describe the study design in the subtitle:

Risk factors for stroke in subjects with normal blood pressure: A prospective cohort study (Li, Engström, Hedblad, Berglund, & Janzon, 2004)

Reading comprehension and understanding idiomatic expressions: A developmental study (Levorato, Nesi, & Cacciari, 2004)

Test-retest reliability of walking speed, step length, and step width measurement after traumatic brain injury: A pilot study (van Loo, Moseley, Bosman, de Bie, & Hassett, 2004)

Effect of soy protein containing isoflavones on cognitive function, bone mineral density, and plasma lipids in postmenopausal women: A randomized, controlled trial (Kreijkamp-Kaspers et al., 2005)

Some identify the source of data in the subtitle:

Use of cognitive enhancement medication in persons with Alzheimer disease who have a family caregiver: Results from the Resources for Enhancing Alzheimer's Caregiver Health (REACH) project (Belle, Zhang, & Czaja, 2004)

Cognitive responses to pharmacological treatment for depression in Alzheimer disease: Secondary outcomes from the depression in Alzheimer's disease study (DIADS) (Munro et al., 2004)

Some hanging titles combine an indicative titles and a subtitled question:

Threat appraisal and avoidance after brain injury: Why and how often are activities avoided? (Riley, Brennan, & Powell, 2004)

The neuropsychology of vascular cognitive impairment: Is there a specific cognitive deficit? (Desmond, 2004)

But sometimes the main title is a question and the subtitle is indicative:

Are there inequalities in the provision of stroke care? A prospective cohort study (McKevitt, Coshall, Tilling, & Wolfe, 2005)

A few hanging titles replace the colon with a dash:

Reversing spoken items—mind twisting not tongue twisting (Rudner, Rönnberg, & Hugdahl, 2005)

Hanging titles are common in behavioral science and medical journals. The titles in the 300-title Medline sample contained 88 hanging titles (29%), most of which could have been written as straightforward indicative titles with no loss of precision.

Perhaps some of hanging titles' popularity comes from an article by Dillon (1981). Dillon compared titles in a group of journals he called scholarly journals with titles in a group of journals he called nonscholarly journals. He found that 72% of the articles in the scholarly journals had colons in the title, versus 12% of the articles in the nonscholarly journals. He also compared titles of doctoral dissertations to titles of articles published by mid-career authors and found a greater percentage of colons in titles of mid-career articles (66%) than in titles of dissertations (16%). Dillon concluded that titles containing colons may be an indicator of scholarship.

Lupo and Kopelmen (1987) evaluated Dillon's conclusions by assessing the presence of colons in the titles of 552 manuscripts submitted to a scholarly journal. Eighty-seven were subsequently accepted for publication, of which 18

(21%) had titles containing colons. Four hundred sixty-five were rejected, of which 81 (17%) had titles containing colons. The difference was not statistically significant, suggesting no meaningful relationship between the presence of a colon in a title and publication of a manuscript.

Hanging titles, although now common, are relatively new in scientific and technical writing, and may reflect a perceived need for eye-catching titles to separate an author's work from an abundance of other titles on similar topics. Some journals encourage hanging titles, apparently in the belief that getting key words up front helps busy readers who are scanning lists of titles in search of articles related to their interests. Day and Gastel (2006), however, comment that hanging titles "appear pedantic, often place the emphasis on a general term rather than a more significant term, necessitate punctuation, scramble indexes, and in general provide poor titles" (p. 44).

Hanging titles encourage redundancy because the first part of the title typically is so general that it provides little useful information about the content of a paper. Hanging titles also create problems for automatic indexing systems, which can be mystified by such double titles.

A hanging title can help get a complex message across with a few words, but straightforward indicative titles usually have more punch and better serve readers who are scanning lists of titles in bibliographies, indexes, or databases. Unless you know that your journal encourages hanging titles and unless you really need a hanging title to do justice to the content of your paper, stick with an indicative title. If you must use a hanging title, write it with a colon, not a dash. Colons are the traditional punctuation for hanging titles.

Series Titles

Series titles are hanging titles in which the main title ends with a numeral showing that an article is part of a series. Such titles are called series titles:

> *The search for common ground: Part I. Lexical processing by linguistically diverse learners* (Windsor & Kohnert, 2004)

> *The search for common ground: Part II. Non-linguistic processing by diverse learners* (Kohnert & Windsor, 2004)

Few contemporary journals accept series titles, primarily because editors believe that every article should be complete in itself. Individual articles in a series often do not provide sufficient information to permit readers to understand any one article without reading the entire series. Series articles are troublesome to readers because their appreciation of an article after the first is compromised unless the preceding articles are available for consecutive reading. Series titles published back-to-back in the same journal alleviate the last problem but not the others. Finally, series articles may give editors (and authors) headaches if, say, the second article is accepted for publication, but the first is rejected.

Length of Titles

Titles for articles in science and medicine have gotten shorter over the years. In the 1800s and early 1900s, titles of articles in medical and scientific journals were long and read much like present-day abstracts, as does this title for a paper published in 1929:

Meningiomas arising from the tuberculum sellae with the syndrome of primary optic atrophy and bitemporal field defects combined with a normal sella turcica in a middle-aged person (Cushing & Eisenhardt, 1929)

Dillon (1981) found an interaction between the presence of colons in titles and the number of words in the titles. Titles with colons in Dillon's sample were about twice as long as titles without colons (17 words versus 9 words). Dillon concluded that the number of words in a title, as well as the presence of a colon, is an indicator of scholarship. But Lupo and Kopelman (1987) disagreed. The titles of accepted manuscripts in their sample of published and unpublished manuscripts were slightly shorter than the titles of rejected manuscripts (5.9 words versus 6.4 words). Lupo and Kopelman (1987) concluded that the number of words in a title, like the presence of a colon, does nothing to improve the odds of publication. They comment, "(a) titular reduction, not expansion, is to be encouraged, and (b) colon-ization of titles is not too important—colons are but small marks of scholarly distinction" (p. 513).

Most contemporary journals discourage long titles. Some limit the number of words or the number of characters in titles. The *Publication Manual of the American Psychological Association* (2010), for example, recommends that titles be no more than 12 words long. Most titles in contemporary scientific and technical journals comply. The average length of titles in our 300-title Medline sample was 12 words. The two shortest were four words long. One was indicative, and one was an assertive sentence title:

Velnacrine for Alzheimer's disease (Birks & Wilcock, 2004)

Donepezil's effects remain uncertain (Royall, 2004)

The longest was 28 words:

Differential time and related appearance of signs, indicating improvement in the state of consciousness in vegetative state traumatic brain injury (VS-TBI) patients after initiation of dopamine treatment (Krimchansky, Keren, Sazbon, & Groswasser, 2004)

Most too-long titles contain extra words that neither establish the topic nor highlight key issues. A common source of extra words is lead-in phrases, such as, "A study of . . . ," "A controlled study of . . . ," "A comprehensive investigation of . . . ," "Effects of . . . ," and the like. Such lead-in phrases usually are dead weight. Another common source of excess baggage in titles is inclusion of inconsequential detail, as in this title:

Effect of posterior temporal-parietal hematoma on orbital frontal chemistry in relation to a cognitive and anxiety state: A combined 1H-MRS and neuropsychological study of an unusual case as compared with 16 healthy subjects (Grachev, Kumar, Swarnkar, Chang, & Ramachandran, 2002)

This wordy title is easily reduced to a streamlined title that concisely conveys the paper's content:

Posterior temporal-parietal hematoma, orbital frontal chemistry, cognition and anxiety.

A title can be too short. A title is too short if it does not give readers the information they need to decide whether to read the abstract or the article. Most too-short titles are too general and do not adequately specify the topic:

Reading comprehension in aphasia

Post-stroke depression

Rehabilitation in traumatic brain injury

Too-general titles leave readers guessing about the point of an article. Is it a research article? A review of literature? A tutorial? Adding detail helps:

Lexical pitch and comprehension of narratives by aphasic adults

Reliability of scales for rating post-stroke depression

Effectiveness of computer-based cognitive retraining for brain-injured adults

Too-general titles cause problems for users searching indexes or databases for articles on a given topic, because too-general titles yield hundreds or thousands of "hits" when their key words are used as search terms. For example, a search of "rehabilitation" and "traumatic brain injury" yielded 3,380 hits. A search of "reading comprehension" and "aphasia" as search terms in a Medline search yielded 175 hits, a much more manageable number. If you want your work to stand out from the crowd, put in the title key words that will uniquely identify the topic.

The main words in a title should be key words that highlight the important content of the paper—the primary topic, the major variables manipulated, and the important theoretical or practical issues addressed, with only as many linking words as are needed to make the title comprehensible. If your title has more than one linking word for every three or four

words, it may be a candidate for simplification. Here is a made-up title with nine linking words and 10 substantive words (and some of the substantive words are not key words because they are too general):

The relationship between the presence of hoarding behavior and the severity of obsessive-compulsive disorder in an adult population

Judicious pruning creates a seven-word title with two linking words:

Hoarding and obsessive-compulsive disorder in adults

Sometimes you may need more than 12 words to specify the content of your paper. Sometimes readability and syntactic quality may make a lead-in phrase such as "Effects of . . . " reasonable. If that happens, go ahead. Put more words in the title. Begin the title with a lead-in phrase. But do so intentionally and not because you are careless or lazy. (Did you notice the lead-in phrase in "Effectiveness of Computer-Based Cognitive Retraining . . . " mentioned previously? We thought the title was too terse without it.)

Syntax

Be mindful of syntax in your titles. Watch word order and be careful where you place modifiers. Faulty word order and misplaced modifiers can create an unintentionally humorous title:

Examining the motor system in the supine position

Pulmonary diseases in humans coming from bird feces

Monitoring patients who wear cardiac monitors around the clock

Neurologic diseases in humans spread by cattle

Excessive alliteration in a title also can make it unintentionally humorous:

Parallel processing and pattern perception in patients with parietal lobe pathology

Hewitt (1957) comments that an unintentionally humorous title is one way to break into print, because even if the paper is rejected, the title will show up somewhere (as in Hewitt's list of such titles). Such notoriety may not, however, help the student along the path to graduation or the scholar/scientist along the way to publication.

Mildly humorous (catchy) titles sometimes pop up in contemporary journals. (Two percent of our 300-title Medline sample were catchy titles. Most were both catchy and hanging.)

Remember that old theory of memory? Well, forget it (Jenkins, 1974)

A psychodynamic perspective on resistance in psychotherapy: Vive la resistance (Messer, 2004)

The assessment of executive functions: Coming out of the office (Manchester, Priestley, & Jackson, 2004)

Capturing attention when attention blinks (Wee & Chua, 2004)

Repetition blindness: Out of sight or out of mind? (Morris & Harris, 2004)

Blink and shrink: The effect of the attentional blink on spatial processing (Olivers, 2004)

Most catchy titles violate the basic requirements of a good title—they do not clearly identify the topic of the paper or the issues under investigation, and they almost always contain unnecessary words. Catchy titles also may cause indexing systems to misclassify a paper. Be careful when you are tempted to put a catchy title on a serious piece of work, because a catchy title risks trivializing the work to which it is attached. Those who take science seriously (including editors) may be put off by a catchy title, and readers searching for significant articles may look twice at your title, but pass your work by as science whimsy. Unless you are sure of yourself, your literary creativity, and your readership, avoid whimsy in titles for serious works.

Abbreviations, Acronyms, and Technical Terms in Titles

Many journals do not allow abbreviations and acronyms in titles. Some permit standard abbreviations and acronyms—those that most readers of the publication will recognize. Most permit undefined technical terms if the terms are recognizable to anyone moderately familiar with the vocabulary of the discipline. A medical journal may allow abbreviations such as fMRI (for functional magnetic resonance imaging), COPD (for chronic obstructive pulmonary disease), and RNA (for ribonucleic acid), and technical terms such as hemodialysis, craniotomy, endarterectomy, and ischemic in titles. A psychology journal may permit abbreviations such as WAIS (for Wechsler Adult Intelligence Scale), PPVT (for Peabody Picture Vocabulary Test), MMPI (for Minnesota Multiphasic Personality Inventory), and ANOVA (for analysis of variance), and technical terms such as discrimination, cognition, mediation, and visuomotor.

Unless you are certain that readers will understand an abbreviation, acronym, or technical term, do not put it in the title of your paper. Be especially careful with abbreviations or acronyms that may have more than one meaning. For example, RT may stand for reaction time, radiation therapy, or reverse transcriptase. SLD may stand for sublethal damage, standard laboratory diet, stutter-like disfluencies, or specific learning disability. PTA may stand for pure-tone audiometry, posttraumatic amnesia, or percutaneous transluminal angioplasty. Although it may be true that the context in which an abbreviation or acronym appears specifies its meaning, if there is any meaningful probability that readers will fail to recognize or will be misled by an abbreviation or acronym, either keep it out of the title or spell it out, as in

Reliability and validity of the KWIC (key word in context) indexing system

Also keep esoteric technical terms out of titles. If your title contains a term that may not be familiar to most readers, substitute a more general term or define it in a few words, as in

Telomeric (chromosomal) mutations in end-stage lung cancer

If a technical term is not a key word, do not include it in a title. But if an abbreviation or a technical term is both important and common in the discipline, and if the journal permits them, then put it in.

Key Words

Databases and indexing and retrieval systems for scientific and technical papers (e.g., Medline, CINAHL, ERIC, PsychInfo) allow users of a database to find titles and abstracts by entering key words as search terms. The retrieval system searches for entries that contain the key words in the title, in the abstract, or in a list of key words provided by the author of a paper. Key words are not always single words but may be strings of several words (e.g., failure to thrive, cause of death, cardiovascular accident, shaken baby syndrome, sensorineural hearing loss, language development). Key words in a title include any words that uniquely specify the content of a paper (key words in bold in the following examples).

Attentional allocation *during the* ***perception of scenes*** *(Gordon, 2004)*

A preliminary study of the ***efficacy*** *of* ***ondansetron*** *in the* ***treatment of ataxia, poor balance, and incoordination*** *from* ***brain injury*** (Mandelcorn, Cullen, & Bayley, 2004)

Key words provided by authors may include key words from the title plus other words that further specify the content of the paper.

Title: *Hypertension and the rate of cognitive decline in patients with dementia of the Alzheimer type* (Bellew, Pigeon, Stang, Fleischman, Gardner, & Baker, 2004)

Key words provided by the author: *Hypertension, dementia, cognition, antihypertensive medication*

Choose key words for your paper so that anyone searching a database for information related to your paper will find your paper and so that your paper is not buried in a mass of works with only general relationship to your work.

Make key words as specific as you can. If you must include a general key word, supplement it with specific key words to minimize the number of tangential or irrelevant works a retrieval system yields when someone enters the key words. Ask yourself, "How would I find this paper in an index?" and compose your title and list of key words to ensure that everyone with an interest in the topic will find your paper. (See also Chapter 13, Getting Published for more information on maximizing the likelihood that interested readers will find your work.)

Here is an example of a Medline search for papers on the effect of donepezil, a cholinesterase inhibitor, on the progression of Alzheimer's disease. Entering general descriptors as search terms yielded large numbers of hits, most of which were not relevant to the topic. Entering "Alzheimer's disease" yielded 43,720 hits. Entering "Alzheimer's disease" and "treatment" yielded 12,980 hits. Entering "Alzheimer's disease," "treatment," and "medication" yielded 693 hits. Entering "Alzheimer's disease" and "donepezil" yielded only five hits. Clearly, the more precise your key words, the more likely it is that someone searching a database with the key words will find your paper and the more likely it is that the citation for your paper will not be buried in several hundred or several thousand irrelevant citations.

Running Titles

Many journals and books print running titles (sometimes called running heads) on alternate pages of published articles. Running titles are shortened versions of the main title. Running titles usually contain from four to ten words, and may contain abbreviations of terms from the full title. Many publishers require that authors include a running title on the title page of the manuscript, and most specify the maximum number of characters permitted for running titles:

Title: *Treatment of depression following myocardial infarction* (Guck, Kavan, Elsasser, & Barone, 2001)

Key words: *depression, myocardial infarction, sertraline, cognitive therapy*

Running title: *Depression and myocardial infarction*

Title: *Lexical diversity in the spontaneous speech of children with specific language impairment* (Owen & Leonard, 2002)

Key words: *specific language impairment, vocabulary, lexical diversity, lexicon, language sample*

Running title: *Lexical diversity in SLI*

Guidelines for Writing the Title

Spend serious time on the title. Remember—more people will read the title than will read any other words in your paper. A well-written title

- gives a concise statement of the topic of the paper in 10 to 15 words;
- conveys the main message of the paper—the issues addressed and the relationships among the issues;
- is indicative, unless an instructor or an editor requires an informative title;
- is fully understandable when read by itself;

- is syntactically well formed but need not be a complete sentence;
- does not contain unnecessary words;
- does not contain nonstandard abbreviations or acronyms;
- defines technical terms that may be unfamiliar to readers;
- contains key words permitting indexing systems to provide appropriate search terms;
- easily compresses to a shorter title for running heads in published work; and
- does not promise more than the paper delivers.

References

American Psychological Association. (2010). *Publication manual of the American Psychological Association* (6th ed.). Washington, DC: Author.

Beck, M. R., Angelone, B., & Levin, D. (2004). Knowledge about the probability of change affects change detection performance. *Journal of Experimental Psychology: Human Perception and Performance, 30*(4), 778–791.

Belle, S. H., Zhang, S., & Czaja, S. J. (2004). Use of cognitive enhancement medication in persons with Alzheimer disease who have a family caregiver: Results from the Resources for Enhancing Alzheimer's Caregiver Health (REACH) project. *American Journal of Geriatric Psychiatry, 12*(3), 250–257.

Bellew, K. M., Pigeon J. G., Stang P. E., Fleischman W., Gardner R. M, & Baker, W. W. (2004). Hypertension and the rate of cognitive decline in patients with dementia of the Alzheimer type. *Alzheimer Disease and Associated Disorders, 18*, 208–213.

Birks, J., & Wilcock, G. G. (2004). Velnacrine for Alzheimer's disease. *Cochrane Database Systematic Review, 2*, 1–28.

Ciccone, A. M., Stewart, K. C., Meyers, B. F., Guthrie, T. J., Battafarano, R. J., Trulock, E., . . . Patterson, G. A. (2002). Does donor cause of death affect the outcome of lung transplantation? *Journal of Thoracic, Cardiovascular Surgery, 123*(3), 429–436.

Coney, J. (2005). Word frequency and the lateralization of lexical processes. *Neuropsychologia, 43*(1), 142–148.

Cushing, H., & Eisenhardt, L. (1929) Meningiomas arising from the tuberculum sellae: With the syndrome of primary optic atrophy and bitemporal field defects combined with a normal sella turcica in a middle-aged person. *Archives of Ophthalmology, 1*(1), 1–41.

Day, R., & Gastel, B. (2006). *How to write and publish a scientific paper*. Westport, CT: Greenwood Press.

Desmond, D. W. (2004). The neuropsychology of vascular cognitive impairment: Is there a specific cognitive deficit? *Journal of Neurological Science, 226* (1–2), 3–7.

Dillon, J. T. (1981). The emergence of the colon: An empirical correlate of scholarship. *American Psychologist, 36*, 879–884.

Dujardin, K., Defebvre, L., Duhamel, A., Lecouffe, P., Rogelet, P., Steinling, M., & Destée, A. (2004). Cognitive and SPECT characteristics predict progression of Parkinson's disease in newly diagnosed patients. *Journal of Neurology, 251*(11), 1383–1392.

Dyson, B. J., & Quinlan, P. T. (2004). Stimulus processing constraints in audition. *Journal of Experimental Psychology: Human Perception and Performance, 30*(6), 1117–1131.

Fischer, S., Siegfried, G., & Trexler, L. E. (2004). Awareness of activity limitations, goal setting and rehabilitation outcome in patients with brain injuries. *Brain Injury, 18*(6), 547–562.

Freed, C. R., Leehey, M. A., Zawada, M., Bjugstad, K., Thompson, L., & Breeze, R. (2003). Do patients with Parkinson's disease benefit from embryonic dopamine cell transplantation? *Journal of Neurology, 250*(3), 1144–1146.

Gil, J. M., Leist, M., Popovic, N., Brundin, P., & Petersen, Å. (2004). Asialoerythropoetin is not effective in the R6/2 line of Huntington's disease mice. *BMC Neuroscience, 5*, 17.

Gordon, R. D. (2004). Attentional allocation during the perception of scenes. *Journal of Experimental Psychology: Human Perception and Performance, 30*(4), 760–777.

Grachev, I. D., Kumar, R., Swarnkar, A., Chang, J. K., & Ramachandran, T. S. (2002). Effect of posterior temporal–parietal hematoma on orbital frontal chemistry in relation to a cognitive and anxiety state: A combined H-MRS and neuropsychological study of an unusual case as compared with 16 healthy subjects. *Journal of Chemical Neuroanatomy, 23*(3), 223–230.

Guck, T. P., Kavan, M. G., Elsasser, G. N., & Barone, E. J. (2001). Assessment and treatment of depression following myocardial infarction. *American Family Physician, 64*(4), 641–648.

Harvard Health Publications. (2004, November). Antibiotics fail to prevent heart attacks. *Harvard Heart Letter, 15*(3), 7.

Hewitt, R. M. (1957). *The physician-writer's book. Tricks of the trade in medical writing.* Philadelphia, PA: W. B. Saunders.

Ishikawa, K., Miyataka, M., Kimura, A., Takeda, N., Hirano, Y., Hayashi, T., & Kanamasa, K. (2004). Beta-blockers prevent cardiac events in Japanese patients with myocardial infarction. *Circulation, 68*(1), 59–67.

Jenkins, J. J. (1974). Remember that old theory of memory? Well, forget it. *American Psychologist, 29* (11), 785–795.

Kohnert, K., & Windsor, J. (2004). The search for common ground: Part II. Nonlinguistic performance by linguistically diverse learners. *Journal of Speech, Language, and Hearing Research, 47*, 891–903.

Kreijkamp-Kaspers, S., Kok, L., Grobbee, D. E., de Haan, E. H., Aleman, A., Lampe, J. W., & van der Schouw, Y. T. (2005). Effect of soy protein containing isoflavones on cognitive function, bone mineral density, and plasma lipids in postmenopausal women: A randomized, controlled trial. *Obstetrical & Gynecological Survey, 60*(1), 41–43.

Krimchansky, B.Z., Keren, O., Sazbon, L., & Groswasser, Z. (2004). Differential time and related appearance of signs, indicating improvement in the state of consciousness in vegetative state traumatic brain injury (VS-TBI) patients after initiation of dopamine treatment. *Brain Injury, 18*(11), 1099–1105.

Levorato, M. C., Nesi, B., & Cacciari, C. (2004). Reading comprehension and understanding idiomatic expressions: A developmental study. *Brain and Language, 91*, 303–314.

Li, C., Engström, G., Hedblad, B., Berglund, G., & Janzon, L. (2004). Risk factors for stroke in subjects with normal blood pressure: A prospective cohort study. *Stroke, 36*, 234–238.

Lin, P. H., Bush, R. L., Lubbe, D. F., Cox, M. M., Zhou, W., McCoy, S. A., . . . Lumsden, A. B. (2004). Carotid artery stenting with routine cerebral protection in high-risk patients. *American Journal of Surgery, 188*(6), 644–652.

Lupo, J., & Kopelman, R. E. (1987). Punctuation and publishability: A reexamination of the colon. *American Psychologist, 42*, 513.

Manchester, D., Priestley, N., & Jackson, H. (2004). The assessment of executive functions: Coming out of the office. *Brain Injury, 18*(11), 1067–1081.

Mandelcorn, J., Cullen, M. K., & Bayley, M. T. (2004). A preliminary study of the efficacy of ondansetron in the treatment of ataxia, poor balance and incoordination from brain injury. *Brain Injury, 18*(10), 1025–1039.

McCusker, J., Cole, M. G., Dendukuri, N., & Bbelzile, E. (2003). Does delirium increase hospital stay? *Journal of the American Geriatric Society, 51*(11), 1539–1546.

McKevitt, C., Coshall, C., Tilling, K., & Wolfe, C. (2005). Are there inequalities in the provision of stroke care? Analysis of an inner-city stroke register. *Stroke, 36* (2), 315–320.

Messer, S. B. (2004). A psychodynamic perspective on resistance in psychotherapy: Vive la résistance. *Journal of Clinical Psychology, 58*(2), 157–163.

Morris, A. L., & Harris, C. L. (2004). Repetition blindness: Out of sight or out of mind? *Journal of Experimental Psychology: Human Perception and Performance, 30*(5), 913–922.

Munro, C. A., Brandt, J., Sheppard, J. M. E., Steele, C. D., Samus, Q. M., Steinberg, M., . . .

Lyketsos, C. G. (2004). Cognitive response to pharmacological treatment for depression in Alzheimer disease: Secondary outcomes from the Depression in Alzheimer's Disease Study (DIADS). *American Journal of Geriatric Psychiatry, 12*(5), 491–498.

Ogawa, Y., Nakagami, Y., Ishizaki, R., Yoshida, H., Parkinson, K. M., Robertson, C. N., & Paulson, D. F. (2001). Heat shock protein 70 (HSP70) does not prevent the inhibition of cell growth in DU-145 cells treated with TGF-beta1. *Anticancer Research, 21*(5), 3341–3347.

Oh, E. (2004). Can we prevent aspiration pneumonia in the nursing home? *Journal of American Medical Directors Association, 5*, 174–179.

Olivers, C. N. L. (2004). Blink and shrink: The effect of the attentional blink on spatial processing. *Journal of Experimental Psychology: Human Perception and Performance, 30*(3), 613–631.

Owen, A. J., & Leonard, L. B. (2002). Lexical diversity in the spontaneous speech of children with specific language impairment. *Journal of Speech Language and Hearing Research, 45*, 927–937.

Rayner, K., Ashby, J., Pollatsek, A., & Reichle, E. (2004). The effects of frequency of eye fixations in reading: Implications for the E-Z reader model. *Journal of Experimental Psychology: Human Perception and Performance, 30*(4), 720–732.

Reinkensmeier, D. J., Cole, A., Kahn, L. E., & Kamper, D. J. (2002). Directional control of reaching is preserved following mild/moderate stroke and stochastically constrained following severe stroke. *Experimental Brain Research, 143*, 525–530.

Riley, G. A., Brennan, A. J., & Powell, T. (2004). Threat appraisal and avoidance after traumatic brain injury: Why and how often are activities avoided? *Brain Injury, 18*(9), 871–888.

Rosner, J. L. (1990). Reflections on science as a product. *Nature, 345*, 108.

Royall, D. R. (2004). Donepezil's effects remain uncertain. *Journal of the American Geriatric Society, 52*(5), 843–844.

Rudner, M., Rönnberg, J., & Hugdahl, K. (2005). Reversing spoken items—mind twisting not tongue twisting. *Brain and Language, 92*(1), 78–90.

Rüegg, S., Bühlmann, M., Renaud, S., Steck, A., Kappos, L., & Fuhr, P. (2004). Cervical dystonia as first manifestation of multiple sclerosis. *Journal of Neurology, 251*(11), 1408–1410.

Samson, D., & Pillon, H. (2004). Orthographic neighborhood and concreteness in the lexical decision task. *Brain and Language, 91*(2), 252–264.

Schlosser, R. W., & Blischak, D. M. (2004). Effects of speech and print feedback on spelling by children with Autism. *Journal of Speech Language and Hearing Research, 47*, 848–862.

Schwamm, L. H. (2004). Statins prevent first strokes . . . and they may improve the chances of recovery after a stroke. *Health News, 10*(6), 10–11.

Siedler, N. W., & Yeargans, G. S. (2004). Albumin-bound polyacrolein: Implications for Alzheimer's disease. *Biochemical Biophysical Research, 320*, 213–217.

Takeyoshi, Y., Hashimoto, K., Fukuda, H., Ishida, M., Arai, H., Sekizawa, K., . . . Sasaki, H. (1996). Oral hygiene reduces respiratory infections in elderly bed-bound nursing home patients. *Archives of Gerontology, Geriatrics, 22*(1), 11–19.

Tjaden, K., & Wilding, G. E. (2004). Rate and loudness manipulations in dysarthria: Acoustic and perceptual findings. *Journal of Speech, Language, Hearing Research, 47*, 766–783.

van Loo, M. A., Moseley, A. M., Bosman, J. M., de Bie, R. A., & Hassett, L. (2004). Test–re-test reliability of walking speed, step length and step width measurement after traumatic brain injury: A pilot study. *Brain Injury, 18*(10), 1041–1048.

van Zoest, W., Donk, M., & Theeuwes, J. (2004). The role of stimulus-driven and goal-driven control in saccadic visual selection. *Journal of Experimental Psychology: Human Perception and Performance, 30*(4), 746–759.

Wee, S., & Chua, F. K. (2004). Capturing attention when attention "blinks." *Journal of Experimental Psychology: Human Perception and Performance, 30*(3), 598–612.

Windsor, J., & Kohnert, K. (2004). The search for common ground: Part I. Lexical performance by linguistically diverse learners. *Journal of Speech, Language, and Hearing Research, 47*, 877–890.

Yang, J., He, L., Wang, J., & Adams, J. D. Jr. (2004). Early administration of nicotinamide prevents learning and memory impairment in mice induced by 1-methyl-4-phenyl-1, 2, 3, 6-tetrahydropyridine. *Pharmacology, Biochemistry of Behavior, 78*(1), 179–183.

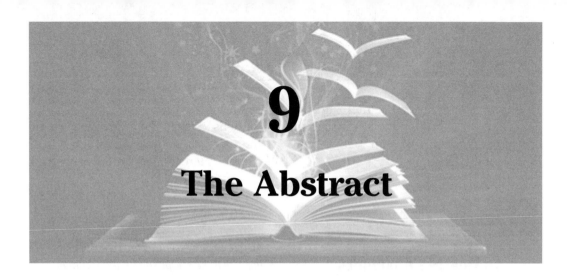

9
The Abstract

"Usually, a good abstract is followed by a good paper;
a poor abstract is a harbinger of woes to come."
—Robert A. Day & Barbara Gastel (2012)

Most scholarly journals print an abstract at the beginning of each article. The abstract is a short narrative that highlights essential information from the article. A well-written abstract permits a reader to get the gist of an article and determine the article's relevance to his or her interests. A well-written abstract does not simply summarize all the parts of an article, but it highlights important elements to help potential readers decide whether to read the entire article. Abstracts of scientific articles also are reproduced in electronic indexes such as Medline, PsycINFO, ERIC, and CINAHL, thus ensuring that an abstract will be seen by many more readers than the article in which the abstract appears.

The form of an abstract depends on the nature of the paper to which it relates and the publication in which it will appear. Format and length requirements differ among publishers. To determine a publisher's requirements, consult the publisher's style guide, read a journal's information for contributors (found on the journal's webpage), or look at recent abstracts in the journal to which you will submit your paper. Abstracts for empiri-cal studies typically range from 100 to 200 words. Abstracts for review papers, theoretical articles, and tutorials tend to be shorter—from 75 to 150 words.

Abstracts for empirical studies typically contain information related to

- the purpose of the study,
- the subjects or participants in the study,
- the method,
- the results, and
- the conclusions and implications.

Those who read abstracts of research articles usually are more interested in the purpose, results, and conclusions than in details about participants or methods, so plan to highlight the purpose, results, and conclusions in the abstract. As you compose the abstract, think of the information readers will be looking for to appreciate the point of your paper, and structure the abstract accordingly. Do not assume that you must squeeze the maximum number of words into every abstract. Readers scanning journals or lists of abstracts mainly want to know if your paper is relevant to their interests and worth reading.

They are not likely to be interested in details, so don't burden the abstract with unnecessary detail, or you risk losing impatient readers.

Kinds of Abstracts

Indicative Abstracts

An indicative abstract is little more than a list that gives an indication of a paper's content. Here is an indicative abstract for a research article on the effects of medication on two types of dementia:

> *The effects of donepezil on adults with Alzheimer's disease and adults with multi-infarct subcortical dementia were evaluated. The performance of participants on a comprehensive test of cognition and mental state was administered monthly for 18 months. Differences between the groups on the test were evaluated . . .* (Krupp, Christodoulou, Melville, Scherl, MacAllister, & Elkins, 2004).

Indicative abstracts give little useful information about method, results, conclusions, and implications. Most journals in the behavioral sciences and medicine do not publish indicative abstracts. Indicative abstracts are more likely to appear in research proposals, pamphlets, bulletins, and nontechnical commercial publications.

Informative Abstracts

An informative abstract does not simply list content but summarizes important elements of a paper. Almost all abstracts for research articles, review papers, theoretical articles, and tutorials are informa-

tive. An informative abstract represents, in condensed form, the purpose and logic of the work as well as salient aspects of its content. Here is an informative abstract for a research article:

> *Seeing a talker's face influences auditory speech recognition, but the visible input essential for this influence has yet to be established. Using a new seamless editing technique, the authors examined effects of restricting visible movement to oral or extraoral areas of a talking face. In Experiment 1, visual speech identification and visual influences on identifying auditory speech were compared across displays in which the whole face moved, the oral area moved, or the extraoral area moved. Visual speech influences on auditory speech recognition were substantial and unchanging across whole-face and oral-movement displays. However, extraoral movement also influenced identification of visual and audiovisual speech. Experiments 2 and 3 demonstrated that these results are dependent on intact and upright facial contexts, but only with extraoral movement displays* (Thomas & Jordan, 2004).

Informative abstracts for research articles appearing in some journals (especially medical journals) are divided into sections that briefly summarize key elements of background (purpose), method, and conclusions, plus a more detailed summary of major results. These extended informative abstracts usually are longer than simple informative abstracts and may give enough information that readers can get a sense of the results and conclusions without reading the article itself. Here is an example of an extended informative abstract from an article reporting on a study of chocolate and tomato extract as antihypertensives. The abstract provides enough detail that readers with only general interest do not have to read the entire article (Chocolate lovers learn from the abstract's conclusion that this study will not help them justify their obsession).

BACKGROUND: Flavanol-rich chocolate and lycopene-rich tomato extract have attracted interest as potential alternative treatment options for hypertension, a known risk factor for cardiovascular morbidity and mortality. Treatment of prehypertension (SBP 120-139/DBP 80–89 mm Hg) may forestall progression to hypertension. However, there has been only limited research into non-pharmacological treatment options for prehypertension. We investigated the effect of dark chocolate or tomato extract on blood pressure, and their acceptability as an ongoing treatment option in a prehypertensive population.

METHODS: Our trial consisted of two phases: a randomised controlled three-group-parallel trial over 12 weeks (phase 1) followed by a crossover of the two active treatment arms over an additional 12-week period (phase 2). Group 1 received a 50 g daily dose of dark chocolate with 70% cocoa containing 750 mg polyphenols, group 2 were allocated one tomato extract capsule containing 15 mg lycopene per day, and group 3 received one placebo capsule daily over 8 weeks followed by a 4-week washout period. In phase 2 the active treatment groups were crossed over to receive the alternative treatment. Median blood pressure, weight, and abdominal circumference were measured 4-weekly, and other characteristics including physical activity, general health, energy, mood, and acceptability of treatment were assessed by questionnaire at 0, 8 and 20 weeks. We analysed changes over time using a linear mixed model, and one time point differences using Kruskal-Wallis, Fisher's-Exact, or t-tests.

RESULTS: Thirty-six prehypertensive healthy adult volunteers completed the 6-month trial. Blood pressure changes over time within groups and between groups were not significant and independent of treatment. Weight and other characteristics did not change significantly during the trial. However, a marked difference in acceptability between the two treatment forms (chocolate or capsule) was revealed (p < 0.0001). Half of the participants allocated to the chocolate treatment found it hard to eat 50 g of dark chocolate every day and 20% considered it an unacceptable long-term treatment option, whereas all participants found it easy and acceptable to take a capsule each day for blood pressure.

CONCLUSION: Our study did not find a blood pressure lowering effect of dark chocolate or tomato extract in a prehypertensive population. Practicability of chocolate as a long-term treatment option may be limited (Ried, Frank, & Stocks, 2009).

Suggestions for Writing Abstracts

Make the Abstract Concise and Specific

Writing a good abstract takes time, attention, skill, and a sense of what readers will be looking for. Keep your potential readership in mind as you compose and write the abstract. The abstract is neither a review of literature nor is it a condensed version of the introduction section of the paper. Most scientific and technical articles are written for a readership that will have at least general knowledge of the domain in which your paper is located, so you need not include material of an introductory nature or describe in the abstract the historical background for the work. Readers will have some interest in the method (to get a sense of the validity of your findings) but will be primarily interested in your findings and what you make of them, so plan to focus the abstract on the results and conclusions. If the method is original and a distinct departure from existing methods, give it more play.

Emphasize what is novel about your work—method, results, arguments, or conclusions—to separate your work from perhaps hundreds of related works on the topic that may exist. Summarize the most important findings and the conclusions arising from the findings, but do not lift material from the paper and place it in the abstract in verbatim form. Do not include material in the abstract that is not in the paper. Do not use the abstract to add to, revise, or correct material in the paper. Do not include incidental findings, and do not imply conclusions that do not appear in the paper. Do not include general statements about recommendations for future work (e.g., "Additional research is needed."). If you are compelled to make recommendations for future research in the abstract, be specific in your recommendations (e.g., "Additional research is needed to determine if the effects of donepezil on cognition are attributable to improved attention allocation or to reductions in anxiety.").

Make the Abstract Comprehensible to Typical Readers

Do not put undefined abbreviations, acronyms, or symbols in an abstract if typical readers may not understand them. Some journals permit undefined abbreviations, symbols, or acronyms in abstracts if the abbreviation, symbol, or acronym is common in the discipline, but others, including those who follow the *Publication Manual of the American Psychological Association*, require that all abbreviations, symbols, and acronyms appearing in an abstract, except for common units of measurement (e.g., mm, kg, sec) be defined on first use. All journals require that nonstandard abbreviations, symbols, and acronyms be defined when they first appear, after which the abbreviation, symbol, or acronym should be used. Do not alternate between abbreviations and spelled out forms either in the abstract or in the paper itself. Spell out the names of drugs, animal species, and standardized tests. Use generic names for drugs.

Here is an abstract for a report in which the authors are careful to define abbreviations that might not be familiar to readers of a neuroscience journal. If this case report were to appear in a medical journal, the abbreviations might be used without definition because most readers who are familiar with medical terminology would recognize them.

We report stroke in a 62-year-old woman who had been on hormone replacement therapy (HRT), estrogen plus progestin, for more than 8 years. She experienced two episodes of transient ischemic attack (TIA), manifesting as right-sided weakness, that persisted for 10–20 min. Magnetic resonance angiography (MRA) obtained before complete stroke, demonstrated severe stenosis of the left middle cerebral artery, without evidence of cerebral infarction. (Inouie, Ichimura, Satoshi, & Ushio, 2005).

Many journals encourage the use of numbers and abbreviations in abstracts in ways that would be discouraged in the body of a paper. The *Publication Manual of the American Psychological Association*, for example, recommends that all numbers in abstracts appear as numerals rather than as words except for those that begin a sentence. In the body of a paper, however, the publication manual recommends that words be used to represent most numbers below 10. Many journals also encourage liberal use of common abbreviations in abstracts, although they discourage such use in the body of a paper (e.g., vs for versus, yrs for years, 1st for first). The next example shows how the use of numerals and abbreviations differs between abstract and body text (text repeated for this example, text in body will be more detailed than in abstract):

Abstract. Participants were tested in 2 1-hr sessions, separated by at least 3 days. In the 1st session 2 tests of recognition memory were administered and in the 2nd session participants' memory for items in the recognition memory test was measured.

Body. Participants were tested in two one-hour sessions, separated by at least three days. In the first session two tests of recognition memory were administered, and in the second session participants' memory for items in the recognition memory test was measured.

Get to the Point

The first thing readers of your abstract will want to know is, "What's the point?" so your first few sentences should answer that question. A good way to do so is with a sentence giving the purpose of the paper.

The objective of this study was to determine the effect of donepezil in treating memory and cognitive dysfunction in multiple sclerosis (MS). (Krupp et al., 2004)

This study compared the copy, cover, and compare method to a picture-word matching method for teaching sight word recognition. (Conley, Derby, Roberts-Gwinn, Weber, & McLaughlin, 2004)

We investigated residual brain damage in subjects who suffered severe traumatic brain injury (TBI) in childhood, and its relationship with declarative memory impairment. (Serra-Grabulosa, Verger, Salgado-Pineda, Mañeru, & Mercader, 2005)

The primary objective of this investigation was to analyze serum concentrations of two biochemical markers of brain tissue damage, S-100B and NSE (neuron-specific enolase), in male soccer players in connection with the game. (Stålnacke, Tegner, & Sojka, 2004)

Several style manuals recommend that writers stay away from descriptive lead-in phrases such as, "This study was designed to assess . . . " or "This report presents the results of a study wherein . . . " which add words to the abstract but provide little information. Many abstracts do, however, begin with such phrases (including many published in journals that recommend against it). If you can begin your abstract without such a phrase, do so, but if the lead-in sentence needs one, go ahead. Do not, however, repeat the title as the first sentence of the abstract—readers have already seen it, and repeating the title adds dead weight to the abstract.

Another way to establish the topic of your paper in the abstract is to begin the abstract with a sentence or two describing the background for your work, if the background would not be obvious to an informed reader. If you choose this approach, keep your description of the background brief and to the point. Provide enough information to permit readers to appreciate the historical, scientific, or theoretical motivation for your present work, but do not try to summarize everything that is in the introduction of your paper. By the time readers finish reading the background information at the beginning of the abstract, they should have a clear sense of where you are going in the abstract and in the article. Here are some examples of lead-in sentences that provide background:

In adult animals and humans, nicotine can produce short-term cognitive enhancement and, in some cases, neuroprotection. Recent work with animals, however, suggests that exposure to nicotine during adolescence might be neurotoxic. (Jacobsen, 2005)

Joke comprehension deficits in patients with right hemisphere (RH) damage raise the question of the role of the intact RH in understanding jokes. One suggestion is that semantic, or meaning, activations are different in the RH and LH, and RH meanings

are particularly important for joke comprehension. (Coulson & Williams, 2005)

The cognitive and neural bases of the ability to focus attention on information in one sensory modality while ignoring information in another remain poorly understood. (deZubicaray, McMahon, Eastburn, Finnigan, & Humphreys, 2005)

The association between white-matter lesions on magnetic resonance imaging (MRI) and the presence of vascular risk factors has been investigated in different populations, and results have varied widely. (Lazarus, Prettyman, & Cherryman, 2005)

If you begin an abstract by describing the background for your paper, be careful not to state the obvious. Self-evident statements such as the three that follow are so general that they give readers no real sense of where the abstract is going. Avoid them.

Depression is a frequent concomitant of Alzheimer's disease . . .

Stroke is a leading cause of death in the United States . . .

Compulsive gambling is a common and highly disabling disorder . . .

A third way to establish a topic at the beginning of the abstract is to begin with salient aspects of the method. Here are some examples:

We conducted an open label pilot study of the effect of bilateral subthalamotomy on 18 patients with advanced Parkinson's disease. (Alvarez et al., 2005)

Using optimized voxel-based morphometry (VEM), we compared the relationship between hippocampal and thalamic gray matter loss and memory impairment in 22 adolescents with history of prematurity (HP) and 22 normal controls. (Giménez et al., 2004)

Verbal and visual recognition tasks were administered to 40 patients with schizophrenia and 40 healthy comparison subjects. (Brébion, David, Pilowsky, & Jones, 2004)

The effects of divided attention were examined in younger adults (M = 23 years) and older adults (M = 64 years) who searched for traffic signs in digitized images of traffic scenes. (McPhee, Scialfa, Dennis, Ho, & Caird, 2004)

Do not include tables or graphs in the abstract, and do not refer in the abstract to a table or graph from the body of the manuscript. Few journals permit tables or graphs in an abstract, and your chances of getting one past a journal or book editor are slim.

Do not cite previously published work in an abstract unless it is a direct antecedent to your present work and your paper is a systematic extension, replication, confirmation, or repudiation of the works cited. Cite previously published work as in this excerpt from an abstract (list authors, with initials before surnames; end with date of publication):

The modular framework of number processing (e.g., S. Dehaene & R. Akhavein, 1995) was applied to study sequential trial-to-trial effects in a number comparison task. (Schwarz & Ischebeck, 2000)

Make the Abstract Self-Contained

The abstract should be a clear, concise, and free-standing summary of the content of the paper. It should supply enough information that readers can get the gist of the paper without reading the paper. Do not refer to material from the paper in such a way that you force the reader to delve into the paper to clarify its meaning. Remember that the abstract will be easier to access than the full paper, so if a concept is not clear in the abstract it might as well not be there at all.

Make the Abstract Readable

Write the abstract in complete sentences and write most of the sentences in active voice. Use verbs rather than nominalizations (e.g., evaluate rather than evaluation, analyze rather than analysis). Use the past tense to describe purpose, method, conclusions, and results. Use the present tense to describe interpretations, generalizations, and implications with continuing relevance.

Purpose: The purpose of this study was (past tense) to determine how well the XYZ test discriminates (present tense) between normal and developmentally delayed participants. (Present tense for discriminates because it refers to a condition that continues into the present.)

Method: Participants were recruited (past tense) from several elementary schools in Gotham City.

Result: All participants performed (past tense) significantly below the cutoff for normal performance on the XYZ test.

Result: Socioeconomic status apparently did not (past tense) affect test performance.

Generalization: Performance on the XYZ test reliably identifies (present tense) children who have (present tense) developmental delays.

Implication: Comprehensive testing is (present tense) vital if developmentally delayed children are (present tense) to be identified reliably.

Maximize Informativeness

Compressing central information about purpose, method, results, and conclusions into 200 or fewer words can be difficult. Keep information density high as you write the abstract. Pack each sentence with information-bearing words, but write the abstract in complete sentences. Do not adopt a telegraphic style in which you omit function words such as "the," "and," "a," and "an." Prune out obvious, general, and tangential information. Avoid empty stereotypic phrases such as, "Group average scores on outcome measures are provided" or "The implications of these findings are discussed." Reduce the abstract to key elements of the paper. Highlight elements that make your work stand out from the work of others. Limit the abstract to no more than four to six major points relating to the paper's primary purpose, important aspects of the method, major results, and major conclusions.

Though the abstract is one of the most important parts of a paper, authors too often write it as an afterthought, just before sending the manuscript off to a journal. Do not assume that, because the abstract is short and because you write it after you have written the rest of the paper, you can knock off the abstract in a few minutes by lifting a sentence here and there from the paper and filling in a few connecting words. A good abstract cannot be an afterthought. Writing an abstract requires time, patience, a sense of what is important to your readership, and willingness to revise and rewrite until it is clear, concise, and fluent.

Guidelines for Writing Abstracts

- Be concise and specific.
- Avoid abbreviations.
- Start with the purpose of the paper.
- Summarize the content of the paper, don't force the reader to look for clarification in the paper.
- Use active voice.
- Use the past tense to describe the purpose, method, results, and conclusions.
- Use present tense to describe interpretations, generalizations, and implications.
- Maximize informativeness: make every sentence count, and avoid empty stereotypic phrases.
- Review the abstract with an editor's eye: does every sentence help reader understanding? If not, it is unnecessary.

References

Alvarez, L., Macias, R., Lopez, G., Alvarez, E., Pavon, N., Rodriguez-Oroz, M. C., . . .

Obeso, J. (2005). Bilateral subthalamotomy in Parkinson's disease: Initial and long-term response. *Brain, 128,* 570–583.

Brébion, G., David, A., Pilowsky, L., & Jones, H. (2004). Recognition of visual stimuli and memory for spatial context in schizophrenic patients and healthy volunteers. *Journal of Clinical and Experimental Neuropsychology, 26,* 1093–1102.

Conley, C., Derby, K. M., Roberts-Gwinn, M., Weber, K., & McLaughlin, T. (2004). An analysis of initial acquisition and maintenance of sight words following picture matching and copy, cover, and compare teaching methods. *Journal of Applied Behavior Analysis, 37,* 339–349.

Coulson, S., & Williams, R. (2005). Hemispheric asymmetries and joke comprehension, *Neuropsychologia, 43,* 128–141.

Day, R. A., & Gastel, B. (2012). *How to write and publish a scientific paper* (p. 57). New York, NY: Cambridge University Press.

deZubicaray, G., McMahon, K., Eastburn, M., Finnigan, S., & Humphreys, M. (2005). fMRI evidence of word frequency and strength effects during episodic memory encoding. *Cognition and Brain Research, 22,* 439–450.

Giménez, M., Junqué, C., Narberhaus, A., Caldú, X., Salgado-Oineda, P., Bargalló, N., . . . Botet, F. (2004). Hippocampal gray matter reduction associates with memory deficits in adolescents with history of prematurity. *Neuroimage, 23,* 869–877.

Inouie, N., Ichimura, H., Satoshi, G., & Ushio, Y. (2005). Cerebral thrombosis in a post-menopausal woman on HRT. *Journal of Clinical Neuroscience, 12,* 109–110.

Jacobsen, L. K. (2005). Effects of smoking and smoking abstinence on cognition in adolescent tobacco smokers. *Biological Psychiatry, 57,* 56–66.

Krupp, L., Christodoulou, C., Melville, P., Scherl, W., MacAllister, S., & Elkins, L. (2004). Donepezil improved memory in multiple sclerosis: A randomized clinical trial. *Neurology, 63,* 1579–1585.

Lazarus, R., Prettyman, R., & Cherryman, G. (2005). White matter lesions on magnetic resonance imaging and their relationship with vascular risk factors in memory clinic attenders. *International Journal of Geriatric Psychiatry, 20,* 274–279.

McPhee, L., Scialfa, C., Dennis, W., Ho, G., & Caird, K. (2004). Age differences in visual search for traffic signs during a simulated conversation. *Human Factors, 46,* 674–685.

Ried, K., Frank, O. R., & Stocks, H. P. (2009). Dark chocolate or tomato extract for prehypertension: A randomised controlled trial. *BMC Complementary and Alternative Medicine, 9,* 22.

Schwarz, W., & Ischebeck, A. (2000). Sequential effects in number comparison. *Journal of Experimental Psychology: Human Perception and Performance, 26,* 1606–1621.

Serra-Grabulosa, J., Verger, J., Salgado–Pineda, P., Mañeru, C., & Mercader, J. (2005). Cerebral correlates of declarative memory dysfunctions in early traumatic brain injury. *Journal of Neurology, Neurosurgery, and Psychiatry, 76,* 129–131.

Stålnacke, B., Tegner, Y., & Sojka, P. (2004). Playing soccer increases serum concentrations of the biochemical markers of brain damage S-100B and neuron-specific enolase in elite players: A pilot study. *Brain Injury, 18,* 899–909.

Thomas, S. M., & Jordan, T. R. (2004). Contributions of oral and extraoral facial movement to visual and audiovisual speech perception. *Journal of Experimental Psychology: Human Perception and Performance, 30,* 873–888.

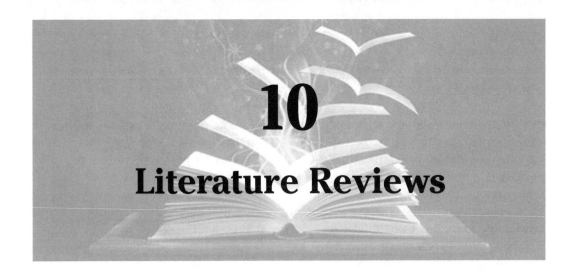

10
Literature Reviews

"The aim of scholarship is to increase understanding, not just accumulate facts."
—M. Tobin (2003, p. 732)

Review articles condense the work of many researchers into a single article. Review articles are useful to researchers new to or returning after an absence from a topic because these articles summarize, and sometimes synthesize, the state of knowledge on a topic. Review articles hold a special place in the scientific literature, and most research databases allow you to limit your search to review articles. Once you've found a relevant review article, its citation list can be a gold mine of useful articles on your topic, as the review author has completed the task of separating the precious from the common articles in the literature.

However, review articles are just the beginning of your search for relevant articles in your topic area. As we saw in Chapter 2 on writing the introduction, you will have to write your own mini-review article on the history and current state of knowledge for your own work. And should you be called upon to write a review article yourself you will need to master the art and science of searching the literature. We will first explore the task of searching the literature faced by all authors, and then the specifics of the structure and writing of review articles.

Searching the Literature

Regardless of its depth and scope, a literature search always involves a trade-off between comprehensiveness and efficiency. Though the ideal may be to find every relevant study that has ever been done, the ideal almost always is out of reach. At some point in the search, the effort involved in searching does not justify the yield—the number of relevant studies identified. No metric tells authors when to end the literature search. Most adopt a pragmatic approach—they begin by searching all the likely and accessible places (e.g., databases, journal tables of contents, and the reference sections of other review articles). Then they search sources that may contain studies not published in journals—technical reports, progress reports, and conference proceedings. They end the search when the yield seems no longer to justify the effort.

You can save yourself much time, effort, and frustration if you keep systematic records of where you searched, the search terms used, the citations retrieved, the sources of the citations, and your reasons for including or excluding articles.

You may find citations for the same article in more than one database, so you should have a way to identify and mark duplicate citations. You also may find the same article published in more than one journal (sometimes under different titles) so you should have a way to group the citations for such articles and mark them as duplicates.

You will search more efficiently if you are systematic in your search for relevant articles. Here are some ways to maximize efficiency without compromising comprehensiveness:

- Use search terms that are likely to identify all relevant articles but exclude irrelevant ones.
- Begin by looking at the key words used to index articles you know are relevant to your topic. Use them to begin your search.
- Add new search terms from relevant articles retrieved in your initial search and try them to see if they are efficient and productive.
- Limit the search to databases most likely to yield relevant works, and begin the search in the place you expect to give the highest yield of relevant articles (e.g., if the review deals with a topic in psychology or behavioral science, begin your search in PsycINFO; if it deals with a topic in biomedicine, begin your search in PubMed.)
- Use the advanced search option, if available. Advanced search allows users to customize the search by restricting it to certain kinds of publications (e.g., clinical trials, English-language articles, adult participants).
- Focus the search by combining search terms with the AND operator (e.g., acupuncture AND treatment AND back pain).
- Broaden the search by combining search terms with the OR operator (e.g., acupuncture OR acupressure AND back pain).
- Specify date limits for the research, if appropriate. If research in the topic area began or ended at a certain time, there is no need to search before or after that time.

Definitions of Review Articles

Definitions of review articles share a common theme:

Literature reviews, including research syntheses and meta-analyses, are critical evaluations of material that has already been published . . . By organizing, integrating, and evaluating previously published material, authors of literature reviews consider the progress of research toward clarifying a problem. (American Psychological Association, 2010, p. 10)

The review paper is designed to summarize, analyze, evaluate, or synthesize information that has already been published (research reports in primary journals). (Day, 1998, p. 13)[1]

---

[1]The words integrate and synthesize commonly pop up in definitions of what a review article is. Integrate and synthesize have related but slightly different meanings, although most thesauri list them as synonyms. The primary meaning of integrate is to bring together and incorporate into a group. The primary meaning of synthesize is to combine so as to form a new (and usually more complex) product.

These definitions suggest that review articles have two primary purposes—to gather information from primary research articles, and to combine the information to produce new insights. The new insights may include

- creating a context that provides perspective on a problem area;
- identifying unifying themes and concepts suggested by primary literature;
- addressing and evaluating controversial issues related to primary literature;
- identifying gaps in knowledge, pointing out methodological problems and inconsistencies in findings of primary literature;
- suggesting new hypotheses, explanations, theories, or models to explain and unify disparate findings in primary literature;
- suggesting how findings from primary literature may be put to use; and
- recommending future research directions and predicting future developments.

Review articles are important tools for organizing information in a problem area and making it accessible to a range of readers, including readers with only passing familiarity with the area. Scientific and clinical journals have published review articles since at least the 1880s, but review articles have become increasingly important as the number of journals and primary research articles has proliferated. More than 20,000 scholarly and scientific journals now publish in excess of two million articles each year. The plethora of primary research articles now produced by a decentralized universe of investigators, laboratories, and institutions makes it physically impossible for most investigators and practitioners in a specialty area to read every article published in that area.

To get a sense of what individuals interested in a specialty area face, we searched Medline for articles published in 2009, using diabetes as a search term. The search yielded more than 17,000 articles. To read all 17,000, we would have to read an article every 30 minutes, 24 hours a day, 365 days a year.[2]

Ketcham and Crawford (2007) estimate that one review article is published for every eight original research articles. Assuming no overlap among review articles and assuming inclusion of all relevant original research articles in every review, one could hypothetically keep up with research in a problem area in one-eighth the time it would take to read the original articles. If the ratio of review articles to original research articles held for articles on diabetes, we still would be faced with reading over 2,000 review articles per year.

Conventional and Systematic Reviews

You will have noticed that review articles come in two flavors; conventional reviews, in which the authors use their own experience and insight to guide their search for material to include in the review; and systematic reviews, where the search methodology becomes an integral and well-defined part of the review. Each

---

[2]Medline is a U.S. National Library of Medicine database containing 5,000+ biomedical and health sciences journals.

type of review article has value in assessing the state of knowledge on a topic, and each has its shortcomings. Learning how review articles are structured and written will help you use them in your work, even if you are not called upon to write one.

Conventional Reviews

Until the 1970s, almost all published reviews were what we now call conventional reviews (also called narrative reviews, traditional reviews, or traditional narrative reviews).

Conventional reviews are historical narratives, usually broad in scope, that trace the development of knowledge, belief, and thought in a field of inquiry. Conventional reviews typically have a broad target audience, including specialists who wish to keep up to date with the findings, opinions, and beliefs of other specialists; professionals in related areas who are looking for coverage of topics peripheral to their area of expertise; graduate students who are looking for an overview of a topic for a paper or report; journalists, consultants, attorneys, and others who are looking for coverage of the literature in a content area related to their purposes; and nonspecialists reading for continuing education.

Conventional reviews are written to provide a comprehensive overview of an area of research. Authors of conventional reviews typically focus on general concepts and broad questions—the "state of the science." They are likely to emphasize influential works—works that have made important contributions to knowledge or have strongly influenced thinking and research in an area. (A work is likely to be thought influential if it is often cited in works by other authors.)

Systematic Reviews

In the 1970s, some members of the scientific community began to question the value of conventional reviews and called for more scientific rigor in reviews. They criticized conventional reviews for lacking a focused question, for using idiosyncratic methods for data collection, for subjective and unsystematic interpretation of findings, and for making recommendations not justified by data.

These criticisms of conventional reviews led to a new approach to conducting and reporting reviews of primary research articles. The new approach, called systematic review, was designed to synthesize research findings relating to issues of diagnosis, treatment, prognosis, and cost effectiveness in medicine and related disciplines. The systematic review approach sought to ensure that review articles respected the same principles of scientific rigor that governed primary research articles.

A systematic review is

> . . . *a review of the evidence on a clearly formulated question that uses systematic and explicit methods to identify, select, and critically appraise relevant primary research and to extract and analyse data from the studies that are included in the review.* (NHS Centre for Reviews and Dissemination, 2001)

The systematic review approach emphasizes comprehensive search procedures to ensure that all relevant studies, both published and unpublished, are found; that procedures for evaluating the quality of studies and for making decisions about inclusion or exclusion of studies are transparent and replicable; and that procedures for synthesizing the findings of individual studies are unbiased.

Meta-analyses are a type of systematic review that evaluate and summarize only studies that use the randomized controlled trial (RCT) design. Randomized controlled trials are the most rigorous designs for determining if there is a meaningful cause–effect relationship between an intervention and an outcome.

Systematic reviews have a relatively narrow target audience—primarily practitioners and policy makers who are looking for answers to questions related to diagnosis, intervention, prognosis, and cost effectiveness. Systematic reviews are an important source of information for people who are concerned with evidence-based practice, in which decisions about the benefits, risks, and costs of an intervention are based on the results of scientifically sound primary research.

Differences Between Conventional Reviews and Systematic Reviews

Systematic reviews and conventional reviews differ in several ways:

- Structure. Systematic reviews have a generic structure that resembles the structure of research articles—that is, sections labeled Introduction, Method, Results, Discussion, and (sometimes) Conclusions. Conventional reviews have no equivalent generic structure. The structure of conventional reviews is more free form and individualized than that of systematic reviews, perhaps because most conventional reviews are broader in scope and purpose than are systematic reviews.

- Style. The style of conventional reviews usually is less formal than that of systematic reviews, although it is similar in some respects to the style in which the introduction and conclusion sections of research reports are written.
- Focus. Systematic reviews usually focus on a specific question (e.g., validity and reliability of a diagnosis, effectiveness of an intervention). Conventional reviews usually deal with broader, more general questions (e.g., the history of a problem area, the development of a theory).
- Sources and selection. Systematic reviews emphasize comprehensive search of the primary literature using carefully described and replicable procedures. Primary research articles are included in systematic reviews based on their quality, which is judged by objective criteria. In conventional reviews, search and selection procedures often are personalized and may be subject to biases, including the author's beliefs, opinions, and attitudes.
- Appraisal and analysis. Systematic reviews use quantitative procedures (usually statistical analyses) for appraising the validity, reliability, and strength of findings in primary studies. Conventional reviews typically base appraisal on the author's subjective judgment about those aspects of findings.
- Conclusions and recommendations. Systematic reviews base conclusions and recommendations on quantitative assessment of the combined results of a collection of primary studies. Conventional

reviews often base conclusions and recommendations on the author's subjective sense of the meaning and importance of individual results, sometimes flavored by the author's personal beliefs.

Conventional Reviews Are Still Important

Some devotees of systematic reviews dismiss conventional reviews because of their presumed methodological shortcomings. It is true that systematic reviews usually are better than conventional reviews for providing objective, impartial, data-based evidence regarding specific diagnostic, intervention, or policy decisions, but not all systematic reviews are paragons of methodological purity. Shoddy search procedures, selection bias, poorly specified, inadequate or inappropriate criteria for inclusion of primary works, and conclusions or recommendations not based firmly on the strength of the evidence may compromise the quality of systematic reviews and conventional reviews alike.

Because of their narrow focus and rigid structure, systematic reviews often do not provide the broad coverage sought by readers who wish to become familiar with contemporary findings, issues, or concepts in a broad domain of knowledge. Dijkers (2009) has commented that systematic reviews' rigid structure and detachment from clinical practice often fail to address values that come into play when practitioners make clinical decisions. He goes on to say that conventional reviews remain popular because their authors do not hesitate to make practical recommendations.

Hammersley (2002) notes that systematic reviews are more precise than conventional reviews because they focus on a specific question—whether a given policy, practice, or procedure works well, or works better than alternatives. She goes on to say, however, that criticizing conventional reviews for lack of focus is unfair:

> *To say that traditional [conventional] reviews are unfocused because they don't concentrate on a specific question is like complaining that a map is of no use because it covers a wider area than the one we are interested in.*

With their expansive scope, personal insights, and narrative style, conventional reviews provide broader coverage of a knowledge domain than systematic reviews. Because they are not focused on a single question, conventional reviews may trace the development of thought in a problem area and may identify the most influential and most useful primary sources in an area of inquiry. Conventional reviews often include theoretical articles, position papers, and primary research articles based on their relationship to a theme or concept, rather than focusing only on articles relating to a specific clinical or policy decision.

> *The historical [conventional] review is an irreplaceable means of tracing the development of a scientific principle or clinical concept; but the narrative thread would be lost in the strict rules of the systematic review.* (Collins & Fauser, 2005)

Conventional reviews usually are written by persons who have extensive knowledge of a topic; in fact, authors of conventional reviews often are invited to write them by book or journal editors. An author's expertise helps to ensure that a review reflects current knowledge, and that theories and conceptual models reflect current thinking. Experts often have practical experience in their area of expertise and are familiar with works related to, but outside the specific focus of the review.

Expertise may taint a review, however, if the reviewer has opinions, points of view, or personal interests that affect selection and evaluation of primary works. Conventional reviews typically require many subjective decisions by authors, including which works to review, what to say about them, and what to conclude and recommend. These judgments are a product of the author's experience, opinions, and attitudes about what is important and what is not in a given field of inquiry.

Structure of Review Articles

Conventional Reviews

Conventional reviews do not have a predefined organizational structure, though most are organized as follows:

- an introduction that announces the topic and places the review in a domain of knowledge and inquiry;
- a rationale that speaks to the importance of the topic and the need for a review;
- a literature review in which the primary literature is summarized and evaluated, and patterns and relationships among findings are described and discussed; and
- a conclusions (or conclusions and recommendations) section, in which the overall pattern,

significance, and implications of findings are described, and in which recommendations regarding continuing research may be made.

In most conventional reviews, this organizational structure is implied, rather than marked with headings. The story told by a conventional review often does not fit neatly into an introduction–rationale–literature review–conclusions format. Consequently, authors of conventional reviews usually organize the review around concepts and topics specific to the literature reviewed, rather than around a generic set of predetermined content labels.

The following example shows the structural organization of a conventional review of research on the use of acupuncture to mitigate depression and anxiety (Pilkington, 2010). The authors included only one generic heading—Conclusions. The other headings denoted topics specific to the review. (However, the first two sections do provide an introduction and the next three make up a literature review and discussion.)

Depression and anxiety

> *Acupuncture theory and practice*
>
> *Clinical trials of acupuncture in depression*
>
> *Clinical trials of acupuncture in anxiety*
>
> *Measurement of biological effects in clinical trials*

Conclusions

The following example shows the structural organization of a more complex conventional review having to do with self-mutilating behaviors in adolescents (Messer & Fremouw, 2008). The first six sections function as an introduction by establishing context and providing background information. The authors organize the literature review around seven models intended to explain self-mutilation in adolescents. The review ends with a future directions section, in which the authors summarize their findings, offer conclusions, and make recommendations regarding the nature of continued research. As in the previous example, the authors used only one generic heading—Future Directions. (This seems fairly typical for conventional reviews. If authors of conventional reviews include generic headings, they are likely to include only one, and that one is likely to be Conclusions, Recommendations, Directions for Future Research, or something similar.)

> (Introduction)
>
>> *Definitions and the continuum of deliberate self-mutilation*
>>
>> *Classification systems and self-mutilation as a distinct syndrome*
>>
>> *Prevalence and incidence rates*
>>
>> *Behavioral and individual characteristics*
>>
>> *Psychological correlates*
>>
>> *Models of adolescent self-mutilation*
>
> (Literature Review)
>
>> *The sexual model/sadomasochism*
>>
>>> *Case studies*
>>>
>>> *Critique of case studies*
>>>
>>> *Descriptive studies*
>>>
>>> *Critique of descriptive studies*
>>
>> *The depersonalization model*
>>
>>> *Survey research*

> *Critique of survey research*
>
> *Longitudinal study*
>
> *Critique of longitudinal study*
>
> *Correlational study*
>
> *Critique of correlational study*
>
> *The interpersonal/systemic model*
>
>> *Case studies*
>>
>> *Critique of case studies*
>
> *Suicide model*
>
>> *Critique of suicide model*
>
> *Physiological/biological model*
>
>> *Between-groups study of the role of serotonin*
>>
>> *Critique of study*
>
> *Empirical study of psychophysiology*
>
>> *Critique*
>
> *Affect regulation model*
>
>> *Between-groups studies*
>>
>> *Critiques*
>
> *Behavioral/environmental model*
>
>> *Empirical studies*
>>
>> *Critique*
>
> *Future Directions*

Systematic Reviews

The organization of most systematic reviews and meta-analyses usually follows a predefined format, which resembles the format of research articles (Introduction, Method, Results, Discussion, and Conclusions). Systematic reviews and meta-analyses typically include these five major headings or their equivalents, but usually add several subheadings (usually in Method and Results) as in the following outline:

Introduction

Method

  Search strategy

  Selection-inclusion criteria

  Assessment of methodological quality

  Data analysis

Results

  Methodological quality

  Data quality

Discussion

Conclusions

In addition to preselected headings and subheadings, most systematic reviews add headings to denote topic-specific content, as in the following example, from a systematic review of the literature on recovery from whiplash injuries (Kamper et al., 2008):

Introduction

Methods

  Identification of studies and assessment of methodological quality

  Data extraction and analysis

    Recovery, pain, and disability

    Prognostic factors

Results

  Methodological quality

  Recovery from acute whiplash

  Course of pain and disability symptoms in whiplash

  Prognostic factors

Discussion

  Course of pain and disability

  Recovery rate

  Prognostic factors

Conclusions

Content of Review Articles

The Introduction

Introductions to review articles range from a paragraph or two (typical for systematic reviews) to several paragraphs or several pages (typical for reviews in psychology and applied science). A well-conceived introduction to a review article serves three purposes. Introductions to review articles, whether conventional or systematic, typically announce the topic and provide context (the opening), offer a rationale, and tell the purpose or purposes of the review. Introductions to systematic reviews, however, usually are more narrowly focused than are introductions to conventional reviews.

The Opening

Openings to published review articles come in several styles, each of which announce the topic and place the review in a domain of knowledge:

- Topic-focused openings announce the topic of the review in the first few sentences.
- Demographic openings relate the topic to social, environmental, or political concerns.
- Historical openings trace the literary history of the topic.

■ Tutorial openings provide information for readers who may not know specialized terminology or technical lingo used in the review.

Not all openings to review articles fit precisely into one of the foregoing categories. Blending of categories is common, with authors mingling, in various combinations, topical, demographic, historical, and tutorial styles in the opening paragraphs of the review.

Topic-Focused Openings. Topic-focused openings predominate in published review articles. Some state the purpose of the review in the first sentence, as does the first sentence from a review of the literature on compulsive overeating (Davis & Carter, 2009, p. 1):

Our aim in writing this paper is to propose, with supporting theoretical and empirical evidence, that compulsive overeating is sufficiently similar to conventional substance dependence to justify its inclusion as an addiction disorder.

Openings that begin with a purpose are surprisingly infrequent among published review articles. Most topic-focused openings begin with a few sentences that place the review in a knowledge domain before announcing the topic.

Here is an opening from a review of literature on "silent" strokes (Vermeer, Longstreth, & Koudstall, 2007); silent strokes are strokes that do not cause overt symptoms. The first sentence places the

review in a broad content area (transient ischemic attack and stroke). The second sentence indirectly announces the topic (brain injury in the absence of overt symptoms):

. . . symptoms and signs of transient ischemic attack or stroke have long defined cerebrovascular disease of the brain. However, the results of neuropathological studies in highly selected populations have shown that vascular disease manifesting as infarcts can result in injury to the brain in the absence of transient ischemic attack . . . [3]

Some topic-focused openings open with several sentences to establish background before announcing the topic, as in the following example, from a review of the literature on posttraumatic stress disorder after the September 11, 2001, terrorist attacks (Neria, DiGrande, & Adams, 2011):

Exposure to the trauma of disasters is common. A national survey in the United States suggested that more than 15% of women and 19% of men are exposed to disasters during their lifetime (Kessler, Sonnega, Bromet, Hughes, & Nelson, 1995). Although the consequences of disasters may include a wide range of psychopathology (Norris, Friedman, Watson, et al., 2002), in earlier community studies conducted prior to September 11, 2001, it had been shown that posttraumatic stress disorder (PTSD) is the most common type of

---

[3]Transient ischemic attacks are incidents of weakness, sensory loss, visual anomalies, or speech aberrations lasting from minutes to a few hours, caused by temporarily reduced blood supply to the brain. The term infarct means death of tissue caused by loss of blood supply.

psychopathology experienced in the aftermath of large-scale traumatic events (e.g., Breslau et al., 1998). The disorder involves substantial functional impairment and is often comorbid with other mental health conditions such as depression, generalized anxiety disorder, and substance abuse. For these reasons, PTSD is the most commonly studied mental disorder in the aftermath of disasters.

Demographic Openings. Authors of review articles on socially significant topics often begin by addressing the prevalence, and by implication, the importance of the topic. The next example is a demographic opening from a review of self-care interventions for asthma (Denford, Taylor, Campbell, & Greaves, 2014). The authors use demographic information to build context and to say why the topic is important:

An estimated 300 million people worldwide suffer from asthma, with 250,000 annual deaths attributed to the disease (World Health Organization, 2007). Despite the existence of effective treatments, morbidity associated with asthma remains high. In the United States, asthma accounts for approximately 1.8 million hospital visits and 500,000 hospitalizations each year (Akinbami, Moorman, & Lui, 2001). The annual economic cost of asthma is estimated to be $56 billion with indirect costs such as loss of productivity estimated at $5 billion (American Lung Association, 2012).

Historical Openings. Historical openings can be divided into two categories, depending on their scope. Some are expansive, taking readers back to the origins of the issues to be addressed in the review—often to times before formal research in the problem area began. Others are focused, taking readers back only to times at which organized research in the problem area began.

Here is an expansive historical opening from a review of the literature on the effects of vitamins and minerals on mood, in which the authors take readers back, first to 1910, then to 400 BCE (Kaplan et al., 2007):

A century ago, the 1910 People's Home Library was a source of in-depth practical knowledge for the populace of North America (Ritter, 1910). Its 500 pages were divided into The People's Home Medical Book, The People's Home Recipe Book, and The People's Home Stock Book. Its medical section guided families at a time when health care providers were not as easily accessed as they are today. . . . Evidence of the role of nutrition in mental health can be traced back even further into antiquity. Hippocrates is often quoted as having said the following in approximately 400 BCE: "Leave your drugs in the chemist's pot if you can heal the patient with food."[4]

Here is an even more expansive historical opening, from a review of the literature on the effects of physiologic stress on the immune system, in which the opening

---

[4]CE in BCE stands for common era, which designates the calendar notation system now in most general worldwide use. Numbering of years in the common era system is identical to that in the Anno Domini (BC/AD) system. The year 400 BCE in the CE system is the same as 400 BC in the Anno Domini system

takes readers back to the mythical time at which time dawned (Segerstrom & Miller, 2004). (Is dawn of time a cliché?)

Since the dawn of time, organisms have been subject to evolutionary pressure from the environment. The ability to respond to environmental threats or stressors such as predation or natural disaster enhanced survival and therefore reproductive capacity, and physiological responses that supported such responses could be selected for. In mammals, these responses include changes that increase the delivery of oxygen and glucose to the heart and the large skeletal muscles. The result is physiological support for adaptive behaviors such as "fight or flight."

Here, in contrast, is a focused historical opening from a review of research on the prevalence of anxiety in persons with dementia, in which the authors take readers back 20 years, at which time organized research in the problem area presumably began (Seignourel et al., 2008). Then they allude to the social importance of the topic by providing demographic information about prevalence:

For the past 20 years, a growing body of literature has examined the assessment, prevalence, and treatment of neuropsychiatric and behavioral problems associated with dementia. Until recently, anxiety symptoms in dementia have received little attention. Anxiety, however, is common in the population . . .

Tutorial Openings. Tutorial openings usually define technical terms and abbreviations or provide specialized information not likely to be known by nonspe-

cialist readers of the review. Here is a tutorial opening from a meta-analysis on how asking research participants questions about their behaviors may change their subsequent behaviors (Rodrigues, O'Brien, French, Glidewell, & Sniehotta, 2015, p. 61). The authors define terms and then describe contexts in which the topic has been observed:

Measuring health-related behavior and/or related cognitions may change the behavior under investigation. This has been called the mere-measurement effect (Morwitz, Johnson, & Schmittlein, 1993; Sherman, 1980) or, more recently, the question-behavior effect (QBE; Ayres et al., 2013; French & Sutton, 2010; Godin, Bélanger-Gravel, Vézina-Im, Amireault, & Bilodeau, 2012). The QBE has been reported for different types of behavior, including consumer and voting behavior (Chapman, 2001; Morwitz & Fitzsimons, 2004; Spangenberg, Sprott, Grohman, & Smith, 2003). More recently, several studies have examined the QBE behavior on health behaviors such as physical activity, blood donation, and cervical screening . . .

Writing the Opening. The opening carries a heavy load. The opening has to engage readers' interest, encourage them to keep reading, and convey a sense of what the review is about.

Sustaining reader interest over the course of a long review requires the skill of a storyteller. A good review pulls readers along without them noticing the tug (Tobin, 2003).

Regardless of how you choose to open a review article, keep your potential readership and the topic and scope of the review in mind. If the review is intended for a readership composed primarily of persons with background knowledge of the problem area, a topic-focused opening should be appropriate. If the review addresses an issue in which social, cultural, or demographic effects are strong, a demographic opening would be a good choice. If the review is intended for a broad readership looking for a panoramic view of a field of inquiry, a historical narrative that takes readers back to the origins of research on the problem (or beyond) may be reasonable. If readers' appreciation of the review's content depends on technical knowledge or terminology not likely to be possessed by potential readers, a tutorial opening may be a good choice.

Readers of review articles can be an impatient lot. If in the first few paragraphs they don't have a clear sense of the topic and why the topic is important to them, they're likely to jump ship. That makes the opening more important than its small size suggests. Spend the time needed to get the opening right. Make it interesting. Tailor it to readers' interests, expectations, and knowledge.

The opening is not an ornament. It leads readers from what they may know (or intuit) about a problem area to the specific issues enumerated in the rationale. Good openings are easy reading and interesting. But they also define the topic, put the topic into historical context, and relate the topic to current issues and concerns.

Don't let creativity entice you into making the opening more expansive than necessary. If the opening spans more than a paragraph or two, look at it critically. The purposes of the opening are to tell readers what the review is about and to prepare the way for the rationale. When you have identified the knowledge domain or problem area to be addressed in the review and have provided enough background information and explanatory material to ensure that readers will not lose their way, you are ready to move on to the rationale.

The Rationale

Published review articles typically follow the opening with a rationale. The rationale section customarily addresses two questions:

- Is the topic important?
- Is a review needed?

Is the Topic Important? Authors of published review articles gravitate toward three justifications:

- Social or economic reasons (e.g., the effectiveness of truancy-prevention programs, the costs and benefits of prostate-cancer screening, the costs to society of chronic obesity). Reviews said to be important for social or economic reasons appeal primarily to a readership composed of practitioners, program managers, and policy makers who are concerned with the costs and benefits of an intervention, program, or policy.
- Political or policy-making reasons (e.g., effects of carbon dioxide on atmospheric temperature, presence of pharmaceuticals in drinking water, economic effects of right-to-work laws). Reviews considered important for political or policy-making reasons appeal primarily to representatives of governing bodies, institutions, and regulators who are concerned with health, environmental, or economic programs and policies.

- Theoretic, conceptual, or scientific reasons (e.g., effects of nicotine on brain chemistry, hereditary influences in schizophrenia, neurochemical explanations of addiction). Reviews considered important for theoretic, conceptual, or scientific reasons appeal primarily to investigators who wish to understand and build on previous work.

These categories are not mutually exclusive; for example, a review of the effectiveness of childhood obesity prevention programs may be considered important for social, economic, policy making, and scientific reasons. Here is an excerpt from the rationale section of a review of the literature on medically unexplained patient complaints. The author frames the importance of the topic in terms of social and economic concerns (Brown, 2004):

> Although many such "medically unexplained" symptoms resolve quickly and spontaneously, symptoms often remain unresolved, causing distress and disability that persists over time. In addition to the suffering and uncertainty faced by patients in this context, the cost of repeated consultation and investigation for these individuals represents a considerable burden to the health care services. This is particularly true in the case of individuals who experience and seek help for multiple unexplained symptoms, for whom health care costs may be up to nine times the primary care average.

Note that Brown went beyond saying that caring for such individuals is costly, but tell us how costly. Keep this in mind as you write a rationale—quantitative data are more interesting and more convincing as evidence for the importance of a topic than are general statements.

Here is an excerpt from a review of the literature on working memory in which the authors relate the topic to scientific, conceptual, and theoretical concerns (Grossberg & Peterson, 2008):

> Intelligent behavior depends upon the capacity to think about, plan, execute, and evaluate sequences of events. Whether we learn to understand and speak a language, solve a mathematics problem, cook an elaborate meal, or merely dial a phone number, multiple events in a specific temporal order must somehow be stored temporarily in working memory. As event sequences are temporarily stored, they are grouped, or chunked, through learning into unitized plans, and can later be performed at variable rates under volitional control either via imitation or from a previously learned plan. How these processes work remains one of the most important problems confronting cognitive scientists and neuroscientists.

Is a review needed? To say that the topic is important is not enough to justify publication of a review article. In the rationale, the author must also tell readers why a review is needed. Though there may be dozens of reasons, the most common are these:

- A mass of primary studies exists, in which the findings are disorganized, unclear, incomplete, or contradictory.
- Studies differ in purpose, participants, procedures, data reduction, data analysis, or conclusions.

- The generalizability, validity, or reliability of findings is questionable or unknown.
- Unifying concepts or theories have not been offered or are inadequate.

Here is a paragraph from the rationale section of a review of literature on psychotherapy and survival of persons with cancer (Coyne, Stefanek, & Palmer, 2007). The authors point out the problematic effects of differences in methods, measures, and participants among primary works:

Evaluating claims that psychotherapy prolongs life after a diagnosis of cancer involves integrating the results of trials that differ in their quality, primary outcomes, recruitment criteria, and sample sizes and in the interventions being evaluated. Integrating these disparate data is a difficult task, and there are no simple solutions.

Writing the Rationale. The rationale should give readers a sense of where the review is going—the key issues to be addressed and the central concepts to be developed. As you write the rationale, focus on key issues and central concepts; do not clutter it with unnecessary detail about specific works. Be careful not to obscure the panoramic view of the topic—that should be the point of the rationale. The best way to keep on track and on topic is to write the rationale with a detailed outline in hand. The time you spend building an outline will save you hours of grief when you sit down to write. The rationale is no exception.

The Statement of Purpose

The statement of purpose for a review article typically is set out in a paragraph or two. Some are short and direct, are expressed in one or two sentences, and focus on a single question, such as this statement of purpose from the review article by Kaplan et al. (2007) on the effects of nutrition on mood:

The primary question addressed by this review is whether our modern scientific literature has provided any substantiation for the folkloric knowledge and early clinical reports about nutrition and mental health.

Some statements of purpose address more than one question or issue. Here is such a three-part statement of purpose from the review of the literature on recovery from whiplash injuries by Kamper et al. (2008):

The aims of the review were to: chart the course of acute whiplash in terms of recovery, pain and disability; identify prognostic factors that are associated with poor outcome; and assess the methodological quality of prognosis studies of whiplash.

Authors of review articles sometimes add information about the organization of the review to the statement of purpose, as did the authors of a review of literature on posttraumatic stress, sleep disturbances, and emotional distress (Levin & Nielsen, 2007):

Therefore, the present review is designed to provide an update of research published since the last major review, focusing on issues of operationalizing the concept of nightmares, estimating the prevalence of nightmares with diverse measurement techniques, explaining the pathophysiology of nightmares, and systematizing the empirical work on personality and psychopathological correlates of nightmares. We organize this research around a model of nightmare formation that takes into account both cognitive–emotional and neural explanatory concepts and that suggests a distinction between two principal factors in nightmare production: affect load and affect distress. Future research directions are also considered at key junctures in the article.

Some reviews add a summary of key conclusions to the statement of purpose, as in this example from Brown's 2004 review of the literature on medically unexplained symptoms:

This article provides a critical review of the different theories purporting to explain the pathogenesis of medically unexplained symptoms, considering both the merits and the limitations of current ideas in this area. On the basis of this review, I argue that (a) different theories are able to account for certain features of medically unexplained illness, but no one theory can accommodate all of the available evidence concerning these conditions, and that (b) no theory provides a satisfactory account of how apparently compelling symptoms can exist in the absence of significant organic pathology. I then describe a novel model that aims to address these shortcomings by reference to contemporary cognitive psychological research.

Writing the Statement of Purpose. Every review article must have a statement of purpose. Most authors put the statement of purpose in the rationale.

Mulrow (1987) comments that it should be at the beginning of the review, which to us means "in the first paragraph or two."

First, a well-conceived review always answers a question. This question should be made clear at the beginning of the review. It should be a precisely formulated statement, rather than a broad or ill-defined question.

Some authors of review articles state the purpose in the opening. Others do it early in the rationale, after the opening paragraphs. Still others state the purpose after telling why the topic is important and why the review is needed. Where you put the statement of purpose depends on the nature of the rationale. Place the statement of purpose where it adds to the clarity, directness, and readability of the introduction. If the rationale is short and direct and lays out a clear path to the statement of purpose, put the statement of purpose after the rationale. On the other hand, if the rationale is long and complex, putting the statement of purpose up front will help readers stay on track.

Do not clutter the statement of purpose with incidental detail. Keep it simple, direct, and on track, and give it in a sentence or two. Do not use the statement of purpose to tell readers how the review will be organized, and do not announce your conclusions and recommendations in the statement of purpose.

The Method

In systematic reviews, a method section follows the introduction. The method section describes how primary research articles were identified (the databases searched and the keywords used in the search), provides the criteria by which primary research articles were included or excluded, and tells how the quality of individual articles was determined.

Because most systematic reviews are written to provide data-based answers to questions about the validity of diagnoses or the effectiveness of interventions, they operate under stringent rules designed to ensure that scientifically sound works are identified and that the search of the literature is comprehensive enough to identify all such works. Authors of systematic reviews typically search major databases of published works, but extend the search to the "grey literature"—works that cannot easily be found in the usual sources (e.g., theses and dissertations, conference proceedings, technical reports, working papers, and preprints). Many authors of systematic reviews extend the search to expert informants (both investigators and clinicians) and to the reference sections of published and unpublished works.[5]

Here is a description of the search strategy used by the authors of a meta-analysis of the literature on the relationship between maternal employment and children's achievement (Goldberg, Prause, & Lucas-Thompson, 2008). The description is a good example of the effort invested in searching the literature for a systematic review or meta-analysis:

One hundred thirteen published and unpublished studies were identified

through searches of the literature. The majority of the studies were identified through broad computerized database searches of PsycINFO, Social Sciences Index, and ERIC, conducted through 2005. The keywords entered, in various combinations, were maternal, mother(s), parental, employment, work, children('s), boy(s), girl(s), achievement, academic, cognitive, cognition, and school. Additionally, the reference lists of retrieved articles, as well as review articles and chapters, were searched manually for relevant articles and chapters. Our own files also were reviewed for preprints, unpublished manuscripts, working papers, conference abstracts, and papers. A handful of relevant studies were identified from the proceedings of national conferences on child development (e.g., the Society for Research on Child Development). Published versions of working papers and conference papers were sought through author searches in computerized databases.[6]

Standard guidelines also require that authors of systematic reviews describe the criteria by which primary works were selected for review, plus the reasons for excluding works from the review. Here is how Goldberg, Prause, and Lucas-Thompson

---

[5]The guidelines for systematic reviews consider the search for unpublished works particularly important because of publication bias—the tendency for journals not to accept studies reporting insignificant or inconclusive results even when those studies are methodologically sound. If studies with positive (significant) results are more likely to be published, they are more likely to find their way into review articles. This bias exaggerates the apparent strength and consistency of positive findings because studies with negative or inconclusive findings have been consigned to the recycle bin.
[6]PsycINFO is a database of scholarly literature in the psychological, social, behavioral, and health sciences. The Social Sciences (Citation) Index is a database of material from more than 2,000 social science journals representing 50 disciplines; it is now part of the Web of Science. ERIC (Educational Resources Information Center) is a database of journal articles, conference papers, books, technical reports, and other materials related to educational research.

(2008) described their inclusion and exclusion criteria:

> *The first selection criterion was that the studies had to test the relationship between maternal employment and children's cognitive or academic achievement. Maternal employment was defined as the mother having been employed either concurrently with the achievement testing or earlier in the child's life. Studies were included if maternal employment was assessed in terms of status (e.g., employed, not employed; full time, part time) or number of weekly work hours. In the overall analysis, achievement was defined broadly to include children's performance on formal tests of cognitive or intellectual development, by academic measures (e.g., school grades), teacher ratings of cognitive competence, or academic rank.*
>
> *The second selection criterion was that the studies must have been published between 1960 and 2005. The year 1960 was established as the starting inclusion point because little or no research on the effect of maternal employment on child development was conducted prior to this year. . . . Studies were excluded when the information provided in the manuscript was insufficient to calculate a measure of effect size and the authors could not be contacted or did not respond to our queries. In all, 45 of the 113 studies retrieved were excluded for the aforementioned reasons.*

Writing the Method Section

You will need a separate method section only if you are writing a systematic review. If you are writing a conventional review, you are unlikely to include a separate method section, though you may choose to describe general characteristics of your search and selection procedures in the body of the introduction. If you are writing a systematic review, include a method section in which you address the following topics:

- databases and other sources searched,
- inclusion and exclusion criteria,
- studies included in the review,
- assessment of methodological quality of studies, and
- data extraction and analysis.

The method section should be an objective, impartial description of procedures. Do not belabor readers with inconsequential details that are interesting to you but do not speak to the adequacy and validity of search, selection, and evaluation procedures. Save your comments and interpretations for the discussion and conclusions sections.

The Results

A results section follows the method section in most systematic reviews. The results section of a systematic review article describes how data from individual studies were aggregated, evaluated, and related to the objectives of the review. Eschleman and colleagues describe their findings on hardiness, a personality trait that is thought to "protect people from the effects of stress" (Eschleman, Bowling, & Alarcon, 2010, p. 277) by organizing their results section to answer the hypotheses that they present in the introduction section:

The results of the meta-analyses for overall hardiness, commitment, control, and challenge are reported in Tables 2, 3, 4, and 5, respectively. In general, hardiness, control, commitment, and challenge were positively associated with other dispositions that buffer against the effects of stressors (Hypothesis 1). For instance, hardiness was positively associated with self-esteem, optimism, extraversion, sense of coherence, and self-efficacy. In addition, hardiness was negatively associated with dispositions that exacerbate the effects of stressors, such as neuroticism, negative affectivity, trait anxiety, and trait anger. Of these relationships, hardiness was most strongly associated with sense of coherence ($p = .63$, $k = 4$, $N = 1,147$), optimism ($p = .58$, $k = 7$, $N = 1,290$), self-esteem ($p = .63$, $k = 14$, $N = 2,610$), and negative affectivity ($p = -.45$, $k = 6$, $N = 3,115$). (p. 286)

The results section also may describe the major results of individual studies and may address the adequacy of design, data analysis, and outcome measures in the works reviewed. In many systematic reviews, however, commentary on design adequacy, data analysis, and outcome measures is placed in a discussion section.

The Discussion in Systematic Reviews

The discussion is the core of a systematic review article. A well-written discussion performs five functions:

- Synthesis. The author groups works according to shared characteristics, summarizes major findings, and shows how findings are related.
- Analysis. The author identifies strengths, weaknesses, common findings, exceptions, and contradictions among primary works.
- Evaluation. The author judges the internal and external validity of conclusions offered by the authors of primary works.
- Integration. The author identifies patterns and traces relationships among findings and points out gaps, ambiguities, and methodological issues affecting primary works. The author may also trace the development of theoretic or conceptual models as they relate to primary works.

The discussion in a well-written systematic review article serves as a quality filter for readers. By screening articles for quality and having well-thought-out exclusion criteria, the author keeps the review on track. By excluding works with major flaws, the author can focus on general issues, patterns, and concepts rather than getting sidetracked into discussing trivial works or works with fatal weaknesses:

The author of a review article . . . sifts through a mass of miscellaneous detail, selecting the most relevant, and omitting trifling reports and ephemeral fads. The value of the article depends as much on the dross and minutiae excluded as the pearls included. (Tobin, p. 732)

Here is an excerpt from the discussion section of a systematic review of the literature on the influence of giving incentives to encourage blood donation (Niza,

Tung, & Marteau, 2013). The authors summarize their findings and conflicting findings, and then suggest possible reasons for the inconsistent findings across studies:

From the few studies that met the eligibility criteria, we found no impact of offering financial incentives on the quantity of blood given. With respect to blood quality, only two studies met the inclusion criteria. One study reported no impact of a gift card on the quality of blood provided. The other study reported poorer quality donations when the incentive offered was a medical test but not when the incentive was a lottery ticket. There was no evidence of motivational crowding-out if operationalized as a lower blood supply when incentives were offered . . . The strength of this review is that it is the first to our knowledge that attempts to examine the evidence for Titmuss' influential hypotheses concerning the adverse effects of using incentives to encourage blood donation. We have revealed the paucity of experimental evidence, as well as different conclusions to earlier, unsystematic reviews. In contrast to the unsystematic narrative review by Goette et al. (2010), based on a mixture of observational and experimental studies, the results of our more robust review do not corroborate their conclusions that incentives increase blood donation.

Writing the Discussion

The discussion section (or the literature review in conventional reviews) should summarize the important works in the problem area, but it must go beyond summarizing to highlight key findings, identify important relationships, and point out methodological weaknesses, unjustified assumptions, and unsupported conclusions. A well-written discussion traces the development of knowledge, thought, and theory in a problem area and critically assesses the reliability, validity, and significance of findings in the problem area.

Imposing order on an unruly literature is a challenge. Only the foolish attempt it without the protection of a detailed topical outline. Organization of the review of literature is a challenge because research on a problem typically does not follow a single path in which investigators approach the problem area from the same direction and study it with the same methods. Instead, investigators often approach a problem with differing attitudes, theories, philosophies, and beliefs, investigate the problem with different methods, and quantify results with different measures.

The focus of the discussion should be on ideas, not authors or dates. Do not routinely begin paragraphs with authors' names or with dates (e.g., "Smith found this and Jones found that." or "In 1990 Smith found this but Jones found that."). Beginning a paragraph with a name and a date suggests that the focus is on who and when, rather than what.

An important benefit of focusing on ideas (in addition to readability) is that focusing on ideas helps to ensure that the review of literature is topically organized —works relating to a common topic are reviewed, discussed, and evaluated as a group. The order in which topics are arranged is not necessarily chronological but should be governed by an underlying theme—the development of knowledge and thought in the research area.

If you have organized the review of literature topically, studies with common elements are grouped together, which will smooth your way as you describe, evaluate, and integrate their findings. Here is how to do that.

Describe common characteristics of each group of studies as they relate to the focus of the review. Do not go into detail about specific characteristics of individual studies unless they clearly relate to the focus of the review. Describe methodology in general terms, emphasizing aspects of methodology that are consistent across studies in a group. Do not include incidental details. Most readers will be looking for commonalities, contradictions, inconsistencies, and gaps as those characteristics relate to the purpose of the review. A well-written review article discusses only those aspects of previous work that are relevant to the theme and focus of the review.

Limit your discussion of problematic aspects of individual studies to characteristics that affect the internal or external validity of the work (i.e., characteristics that influence the replicability and generalization). Focus the discussion of reviewed works on parallel findings, inconsistent or conflicting findings, and gaps in knowledge. Emphasize parallel findings among studies with differing methodologies, because parallelism under differing conditions suggests a strong effect. Point out conflicting findings among studies with the same or similar methodologies, because disagreement under such conditions suggests a weak effect.

Works relating to a topic or subtopic may be organized chronologically if chronologic order conveys the evolution of knowledge and thought in the topic domain. When scientific progress on a topic reflects a slow accumulation of knowledge, with investigators building on the findings of previous investigators, chronological order may be a good way to portray the process. Chronological order has two advantages under these conditions. First, chronological order resembles the pattern to which readers are accustomed in other kinds of reading, such as novels and news articles. Second, the most recent (and presumably most significant) works are presented last, which gives them greater prominence and makes them more likely to be remembered by readers. But if the growth of knowledge about a topic is not orderly—if there are gaps, inconsistencies, or contradictions, or if early works remain influential in current times, chronologic organization may not be appropriate. Then, topical organization is a better choice.

Conclusions (Conclusions and Recommendations)

In the conclusions section of a review article, the author summarizes the central findings of the review and relates the central findings to the purpose or purposes of the review. If the review is a systematic review, the author usually addresses the implications of the findings for clinical practice. Many authors of review articles close the discussion section with recommendations for how research on the topic should proceed, as does Pilkington (2010):

Results of trials in acute short-term anxiety situations appear promising but the relevance to chronic conditions such as generalised anxiety disorder is also unclear. Studies assessing whether acupuncture is efficacious as an adjunct to other established treatment approaches may also be valuable.

Writing the Conclusions Section

Confine your conclusions to the central findings of the review. Do not comment on incidental findings or methodological faults of individual studies. Do not engage in empty speculation. Base your conclusions firmly on the central findings and show how your conclusions relate to those findings. Tell what is noteworthy about the evidence provided by the reviewed works.

Close the conclusions section with a take-home message—a paragraph or two that summarizes the key findings, conclusions, and recommendations of the review. Do not make the take-home message simply a rehash of previous work, but use it to offer new insights, new ideas, and new ways of thinking about the topic or the problem by unifying, integrating, and explaining controversial, contradictory, or ambiguous findings. The take-home message should help readers decide what to do with the information provided in the review. It should leave readers with a clear sense of what is known, what is believed, and what is yet to be learned in the problem area, and it should encourage readers to apply the findings of the review to their own interests and purposes.

References

American Psychological Association. (2010). *Publication manual of the American Psychological Association* (6th ed.). Washington DC: Author.

Brown, R. J. (2004). Psychological mechanisms of medically unexplained symptoms: An integrative conceptual model. *Psychological Bulletin, 130*, 790–812.

Collins, J. A., & Fauser, B. C. J. M. (2005). Balancing the strengths of systematic and narrative reviews. *Human Reproduction Update, 11*, 103–104.

Coyne, J. C., Stefanek, M., & Palmer, S. C. (2007). Psychotherapy and survival in cancer: The conflict between hope and evidence. *Psychological Bulletin, 133*, 367–394.

Davis, C., & Carter, J. C. (2009). Compulsive overeating as an addiction disorder. A review of theory and evidence. *Appetite, 53*, 1–8.

Day, R. (1998). *How to write and publish a scientific paper* (5th ed.). Phoenix, AZ: Oryx Press.

Denford, S., Taylor, R., Campbell, J., & Greaves, C. (2014). Effective behavior change techniques in asthma self-care interventions: Systematic review and meta-regression. *Health Psychology, 33*, 577–587.

Dijkers, M. P., and Task Force on Systematic Reviews and Guidelines. (2009). The value of traditional reviews in the era of systematic review. *American Journal of Physical Medicine and Rehabilitation, 88*, 423–430.

Eschleman, K., Bowling, N., & Alarcon, G. (2010). A meta-analytic examination of hardiness. *International Journal of Stress Management, 17*, 277–307.

Goldberg, W. A., Prause, J., & Lucas-Thompson, R. (2008). Maternal employment and children's achievement in context: A meta-analysis of four decades of research. *Psychological Bulletin, 134*, 77–108.

Grossberg, S., & Peterson L. R. (2008). Laminar cortical dynamics of cognitive and motor working memory, sequence learning and performance: Toward a unified theory of how the cerebral cortex works. *Psychological Review, 115*, 677–732.

Hammersley, M. (2002). *Systematic or unsystematic, is that the question? Some reflections on the science, art, and practice of reviewing research evidence.* Public Health Steering Group, Health Management Agency, United Kingdom: October (p. 5). Retrieved from www.nice.org.uk

Kamper, S. J., Rebbeck, T. J., Maher, C. G., McAuley, J. H., & Sterling, M. (2008). Course and prognostic factors of whiplash: A systematic review and meta-analysis. *Pain, 138*, 617–629.

Kaplan, B. J., Crawford, S. G., Field, C. J., & Simpson, J. S. (2007). Vitamins, minerals, and mood. *Psychological Bulletin, 133,* 747–760.

Ketcham, C., & Crawford, J. (2007). The impact of review articles. *Laboratory Investigation, 87,* 1174–1185.

Levin, R., & Nielsen, T. A. (2007). Disturbed dreaming, posttraumatic stress disorder, and affect distress: A review and neurocognitive model. *Psychological Bulletin, 133,* 482–528.

Messer, J. M., & Fremouw, W. J. (2008). A critical review of explanatory models for self-mutilating behavior in adolescents. *Clinical Psychology Review, 28,* 162–178.

Mulrow, C. D. (1987). The medical review article: State of the science. *Annals of Internal Medicine, 106,* 487.

Neria, Y., DiGrande, L., & Adams, B. (2011). Posttraumatic stress disorder following the September 11, 2001, terrorist attacks: A review of the literature among highly exposed populations. *American Psychologist, 66,* 429–446.

NHS Centre for Reviews and Dissemination. (2001). *CRD guidelines for those carrying out or commissioning reviews* (2nd ed.). York, UK: University of York.

Niza, C., Tung, B., & Marteau, T. (2013). Incentivizing blood donation: Systematic review and meta-analysis to test Titmuss' hypotheses. *Health Psychology, 32,* 941–949.

Pilkington, K. (2010). Anxiety, depression, and acupuncture: A review of the clinical research. *Autonomic Neuroscience: Basic and Clinical, 157*(1–2, Special issue), 91–95.

Rodrigues, A., O'Brien, N., French, D., Glidewell, L., & Sniehotta, F. (2015). The question-behavior effect: Genuine effect or spurious phenomenon? A systematic review of randomized controlled trials with meta-analyses. *Health Psychology, 34,* 61–78.

Segerstrom, S. C., & Miller, G. E. (2004). Psychological stress and the human immune system: A meta-analytic study of 30 years of inquiry. *Psychological Bulletin, 130,* 601–630.

Seignourel, P. J., Kunik, M. E., Snow, L., Wilson, N., & Stanley, M. (2008). Anxiety in dementia: A critical review. *Clinical Psychology Review, 28,* 1071–1083.

Tobin, M. J. (2003). Writing a review article for AJRCCM. *American Journal of Respiratory and Critical Care Medicine, 168,* 732–734.

Vermeer, S. E., Longstreth, W. T., & Koudstall, P. J. (2007). Silent brain infarcts: A systematic review. *Lancet Neurology, 6,* 611–619.

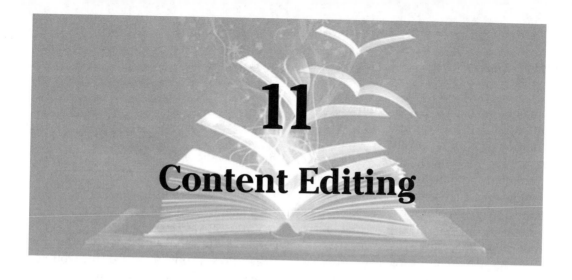

11

Content Editing

*"I have rewritten—often several times—every word I have
ever published. My pencils outlast their erasers."*

—Vladimir Nabokov

The first draft is complete. You have covered the major ideas, and the progression of ideas makes sense. You may think that the hard work is behind you—that rewriting a sentence here and there, changing an occasional word or phrase, and correcting scattered errors in spelling and punctuation will yield a manuscript that will draw compliments from colleagues, plaudits from editors, and admiring comments from tenure committees. Not likely. Unless you are very skilled or very fortunate, you are in for more work. That work is called editing. Successful writers typically spend more time at editing than at writing:

*I can't write five words but that
I change seven.* (Dorothy Parker)

Impatient writers typically underestimate the time and effort needed for editing. They skip outlining and jump into the first draft as soon as they have a fuzzy idea of what they want to say. They struggle through a draft without a clear sense of direction. By the time they finish, they are exhausted and want nothing more than to get the paper behind them. They

do a perfunctory read-through, repair the most obvious faults, and type the result as a final draft. The result is a poorly written paper that only those who are compelled by their work responsibilities (instructors, thesis advisors) will struggle through.

Producing a publishable paper from a first draft requires time, discipline, patience, and diligence. It's a huge help if the first draft is based on a detailed outline. The detailed outline helps to ensure that the organization of the first draft is at least passable, that there are no gaping holes in the progression of ideas, that the progression of ideas makes sense, and that verbal flights of fancy are minimized. Even so, much work remains—editing a first draft into a final draft.

Here is an overview of how most book publishers organize the editing process (more on the publishing process in Chapter 13, Getting Published). Most move a manuscript through three editing stages. A content editor evaluates the manuscript to ensure that it is well organized; that all important information is present; and that the manuscript is free of tangential or digressive material, errors, inconsistency, faulty logic, and vague or unsupported assumptions or points of view. A copy editor evaluates the manuscript for appropriate style, word usage, grammar, and punctuation. A proofreader reviews the typeset copy (called a proof copy or page proofs) and corrects errors in spelling, punctuation, and format (a process called line editing).

The editorial approach we use and recommend resembles that of book publishers. We separate manuscript editing into content editing and copy editing. We divide content editing into three parts —review, markup, and revision—because they require different mind-sets. In review, one adopts the mind-set of an average reader who wants to get the overall point (gist) of what is written. In markup one adopts the mind-set of an editor who is looking for faults that affect the integrity and readability of a manuscript, and and fixing them. In revision, one adopts the mind-set of (dispassionate) authors who know their purpose and who can align what is written with what is intended.

Moving From the Writer's Mind to the Editor's Mind

It will be difficult (and usually impossible) to see what you have written from a reader's or an editor's point of view if the ideas you had in mind as you wrote the first draft are still in your mind as you move into review, markup, and revision. When you are in the afterglow of creation, it's easy to mistake what is in one's mind for what is on the paper. It's easy not to notice that some ideas are underspecified, that others are overdeveloped, that transitions among ideas are weak or missing, and that ideas that seemed perfectly clear when you wrote them actually are muddled and confusing.

Keep the writer from whispering into the ear of the editor as you review and revise. Clear your mind of the peripheral thinking that went into the first draft. Give the thoughts you had in mind as you put ideas on paper time to fade from memory. Forget about what you have written for a few days. Print the first draft. Double-space it and leave wide margins—at least one inch all around. Then put it out of sight. Take a break. Call your mother. Weed the garden. Go to a movie. Don't return to the first draft until you can see it with the eyes of a dispassionate editor.

Review

Don't try to find and correct every fault in one pass through the draft. On that path madness lies. Break content editing into manageable parts. Begin by reading through the draft from beginning to end to get a general sense of its content, organization, and readability. Mark major faults that affect the global characteristics of text that determine its overall unity and sense of purpose. Do not concern yourself with characteristics such as word choice, sentence format, or grammar. As you review, focus on five general qualities:

- Organization. Is the organization of the paper clear and easy to follow?
- Purpose. Is the point or purpose of the paper and of each section clear?
- Completeness. Are all the important ideas covered?
- Emphasis. Do some ideas get too much or too little emphasis?
- Directness. Do some ideas seem tangential or digressive?

The purpose of review is to get a sense of content, organization, and readability. To keep review painless and effective, relinquish the "keep-the-words-flowing" mind-set of the writer and take up the "does-this-make-sense" mind-set of an editor. Read the manuscript through from beginning to end without stopping. Get a sense of how well the manuscript communicates what you want readers to know. Keep your eyes and mind moving. Don't look for, mark, or repair flaws, but try for a general sense of which parts of the manuscript need editorial work.

Markup

Now work your way through the draft paragraph by paragraph. Mark faults that affect the manuscript's unity and sense of purpose. Make liberal use of notes and comments to guide yourself through revision:

- Mark material that seems tangential or digressive.
- Mark locations where transitions are weak or nonexistent.
- Mark ideas that seem vague and do not flow naturally from what precedes them.
- Mark ideas that seem to be getting too much or too little emphasis.
- Bracket material that seems out of place. If you have a sense of where to relocate the material, indicate the new location with a marginal note.
- Add missing headings and subheadings.

Don't fret about minor faults (word choice, sentence structure, and the like). Minor faults that you repair during markup may be removed when you get to revision.

When you finish markup, the draft may look a mess, but you have a guide that will save you time and misery when you revise.

Revision

Now work through the marked-up manuscript. Delete, rewrite, relocate, and revise according to the markup. Expect to do a lot of cutting. Writers usually include more in a first draft than is needed to communicate what they have to say. Minor points the writer knows well get attention whereas major points the writer is less familiar with are neglected. Sometimes an idea seems so compelling that the writer works it in, even though it has little to do with the point of the paper. The free-ranging writer's mind sometimes leads writers on "oh that reminds me" excursions away from the story they should be telling. First drafts almost always are cluttered with verbal brush piles that need clearing.

Move out-of-place material to a location that suits your purpose and that makes sense to readers. Clarify vague ideas. Prop up underspecified ideas, and move overspecified ones further into the background. Strengthen weak transitions. Cut material that is not necessary. If you cannot bear to hit the "delete" button, then cut the material, paste it to the end of the document, and label it as "not used." Unless it is a true treasure, you will find it easy to delete later. Don't edit sentences, change punctuation, or correct spelling errors. That's copy editing.

Keep moving. The draft you create from the marked-up first draft will not be the final draft, so don't work for perfection. Work for a draft that is shorter, better organized, and more readable than the first draft—a draft that you will review, revise, and edit to bring it closer to a final draft. You don't have to get it right the first time (or the second, or the third).

Don't skimp on content editing. Keep at it until you are satisfied with the organization, readability, and logical integrity of the manuscript. That usually requires several cycles of review and revision. When you are satisfied, print it out (double-spaced, with wide margins) and put it away for a day or two to clear your mind of the thoughts that were there as you edited content. When you next take up the manuscript, you will be looking at the draft with the eyes of a copy editor.

editor for mark-up, and an author for revision.

- Review the organization, purpose, completeness, emphasis, and directness.
- Mark up places where the arguments are tangential, vague, or out of place.
- Take a break: Call your mother. Good content editing takes time.
- Revise by deleting, rewording, or moving ideas that you highlighted during markup.

Guidelines for Content Editing

- Change your mind-set to match the task at hand: a reader for review, an

Reference

McPherson Shilling, L., & Fuller, L. (1997). *Dictionary of quotations in communications* (p. 198). Westport, CT: Greenwood.

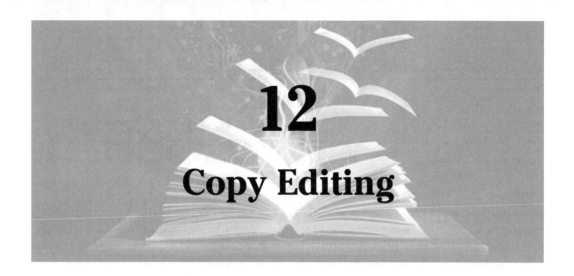

12
Copy Editing

"Editing might be a bloody trade, but knives aren't the exclusive property of butchers. Surgeons use them too."

—Blake Morrison (2005)

You are ready to take the content-edited draft another step toward a completed manuscript. If you have done an adequate job of content editing, ideas that were redundant, tangential, or irrelevant are gone, and the remaining ideas are logically organized and relate directly to the purpose. Transitions from paragraph to paragraph and section to section give unity. Headings and subheadings are in place. Now that you have a content-edited draft, your editorial focus changes from ideas to words, to sentences, and to the relationships among sentences.

Removing Clutter

If you are like most writers (even experienced, successful writers), your first drafts are littered with verbal clutter—words, phrases, and sentences that have little or nothing to do with what you have to say, but creep in when you are preoccupied with getting your ideas down on paper. Content editing removed the brush piles of extraneous material from the first draft,

what remains are isolated words and phrases we habitually use, which flow onto the page without thought or effort. The clutter becomes visible only when we return with the analytic eye of the copy editor.

The purpose of copy editing is to make a manuscript concise, clear, and comprehensible. Clutter provides ideal cover for vague, ambiguous, and awkward writing, so always begin copy editing by finding and cutting clutter. Get rid of the clutter before you edit specific aspects of text such as sentence structure, word choice, grammar, spelling, and punctuation. If you edit specifics before you get rid of clutter, you risk wasting your time and energy editing clutter that you cut later. So begin copy editing by cutting out the clutter.

Anticipatory Expletive Constructions

A good way to vanquish clutter is to prune wordy sentence beginnings—a common source of clutter. Anticipatory expletive constructions are common sources of wordy sentence beginnings.

The word expletive comes from a Latin word meaning "to fill." Expletive, in grammarian lingo, denotes a word or phrase that conveys no independent meaning but adds emphasis or contributes to the rhythm of a sentence. One kind of expletive, called anticipatory expletive construction, is a common source of cluttered sentences in science writing. An anticipatory expletive construction consists of a filler word such as "it," "that," "there," or "this" which begins a sentence and acts as a placeholder for the deferred subject, as in

There are several potential sources for this effect.

The filler word is linked to the deferred subject with a verb such as "is," "are," or "seems," and a connecting word such as "that," "to," "which," "for," or "who." In the following example, the expletive "it" anticipates the deferred subject, "rule."

It is a rule that the word data is plural.

Expletive constructions have legitimate uses. They may emphasize a particular idea in a sentence:

It was Jones who first identified the issue.

Expletive constructions are reasonable when no other subject seems appropriate:

There are many procedures for measuring the readability of printed texts.

Expletive constructions improve readability when the true subject is a long phrase or clause:

There are legitimate reasons for questioning the role of pentathiamine in moderating the biochemical effects of metaclavinol on the permeability of cell membranes.

Carefully used expletive constructions highlight important information and enhance comprehension. But needless expletive constructions add unneeded words. Unnecessary expletive constructions usually begin with "it" and end with "that."

It was found that younger participants had quicker reaction times than older participants.

It sometimes happened that participants became aware of the purpose of the experiment.

It appears that Moody and Williams were unaware of Crandall's findings.

Eliminating unneccesary expletive constructions strengthens sentences by making the true subject the grammatical subject, and by eliminating the extra words required by the expletive construction:

Younger participants had quicker reaction times than older participants.

Some participants became aware of the purpose of the experiment.

Moody and Williams apparently were unaware of Crandall's findings.

Why are unnecessary expletive constructions common in scientific and academic writing? Some writers include them from habit or because they have seen them in published work. Instead of beginning a sentence with the true subject and verb, they tack on phrases that add unneeded words and obscure the point of the sentence:

It has long been known that . . .

It goes without saying that . . .

There is general agreement that . . .

Some writers use expletive constructions to add luster to prosaic statements:

It has long been known that obesity is a major public health problem.

It is important to note that Carmody and James were the first to report this effect.

There can be little doubt that increasing the duration of treatment will result in improvements in outcome.

Some writers use expletive constructions to hedge when they wish to gloss over troublesome facts. Expletive constructions with "seems," "appears," and "may" are particularly common in science writing:

It may be that larger samples are needed.

It would appear that the hypothesis was not confirmed.

Some writers use expletive constructions to duck responsibility when what they have to say may be unpleasant or controversial:

There is reason to believe that the strength of the treatment effect was exaggerated by the authors' choice of outcome measures.

It can be said that Plotkin's model does not explain these phenomena.

Learn to recognize expletive constructions in your writing. When you find one, look at it carefully. Does the thought or the rhythm of the sentence require it? Does it call attention to an idea in the sentence? Does it add emphasis? If you answer "no" to each question, the construction is excess baggage. Get rid of it.

Watered-Down Verbs

When you have gotten rid of unnecessary expletive constructions, turn your attention to verbs. Verbs are the hardest-working sentence elements because they carry the action. But some verbs work harder than others.

Verbs such as "write," "lunge," "build," and "weep" express specific actions and create mental images in readers' minds. Style manuals refer to them as strong verbs. Other verbs express static states such as being (is, are, was, were), possessing (have, had), doing (do, does, did), getting (get, got), and using (use, used). Style manuals refer to verbs expressing static states as weak verbs. Static-state verbs cannot stand alone but must be propped up by adverbs, prepositional phrases, or both:

The authors were of the opinion that the results supported their hypotheses.

Each participant had the option of leaving the study at any time.

Their results had the appearance of reliability.

Getting rid of weak verbs adds luster to sentences, clarifies syntax, and lessens word glut:

The authors claimed that the results supported their hypotheses.

Participants could leave the study at any time.

Their results appeared reliable.

Nominalizations

Weak verbs often walk hand in hand with what grammarians call *nominalizations*. Nominalizations are nouns made from verbs or adjectives. Verbs are nominalized by adding suffixes, such as *-tion*, *-ance*, *-ment*, and the like, to a verb. Adjectives are nominalized by adding suffixes, such as *-acy*, *-ility*, *-ity*, *-ment*, or *-ness*, to the base adjective. Nominalizations can be useful (more on this later), but too often nominalizations weaken sentences by smothering strong words and adding unnecessary words.

Nominalized Verbs

Nominalized verbs weaken the action of a sentence by placing an abstract (weak) verb in the verb position and adding a (usually pretentious) nominal. Nominals often spawn heavy-handed sentences because a new verb must be added to replace the nominalized verb, and a preposition (usually "of," but sometimes "for," "to," or "that") must be added to fit the hodgepodge into the sentence. Consider the following examples. (The nominals are in boldface.)

Examination of the results resulted in revision of our conclusions.

Calculation of each participant's change score was accomplished before analysis of the group results was begun.

Specification of criteria for participant selection is required.

Identification of potential sources of participants was accomplished before implementation of the study was undertaken.

The nominals in these examples shift the action of the sentence to weak verbs ("resulted," "was accomplished," "is required," "was undertaken"). Getting rid of the nominals creates more energetic and more interesting sentences with clearer syntax and greater energy:

We examined the results and revised our conclusions.

We calculated each participant's change score before we analyzed the group results.

Specify the criteria by which participants are selected.

We identified potential sources of participants before we began the study.

Nominalizations are a common source of ponderous style in scientific and academic writing. Nominalizations can squeeze life from sentences by replacing action verbs such as "collect," "measure," and "calculate" with inert nouns such as "collection," "measurement," and "calculation." The action then must be carried by weak verbs such as "is," "was," "do," and "give," or their fat cousins ("accomplish," "administer," "carry out," "complete," "create," "enable," "execute," "make," "provide," and the like), and a preposition or a relative clause must be added to link the nominalization to the sentence. The clutter adds to the reader's workload by loading memory with useless information and by obscuring relationships among sentence elements.

Some nominalizations do not add a suffix to the base verb but have the same odious effects on sentences. Find the nominalizations in these two sentences. The nominalizations do not have suffixes:

I found no contaminants when I took a sample of the filtered solution.

Albertson and Binney wrote a review of the literature in this area.

"Sample" and "review" are nominalizations. Like other nominalizations, they replace a verb with a noun and force the writer to add another verb to take the place of the nominalized verb, plus an article and a preposition to link the concoction to the rest of the sentence. Changing the nominalizations to verbs streamlines the sentences:

I found no contaminants when I sampled the filtered solution.

Albertson and Binney reviewed the literature in this area.

"Sample," "review," "report," and "request" often appear in science writing, and because their nominal forms are the same as their verb forms, they can evade detection unless the writer recognizes the tell-tale weak verb + article + nominal syntax giving away their presence.

Some nominalizations are built around a synonym or near synonym for a nominalized verb:

In the next section we give an account of the procedures used to standardize the test.

Osborne's comments suggested that he was of the same opinion as Fitzgerald.

Getting rid of the nominalizations slims and strengthens the sentences:

In the next section we describe the procedures used to standardize the test.

Osborne's comments suggested that he agreed with Fitzgerald.

Nominalized Adjectives

Nominalized adjectives are less common than nominalized verbs in scientific and academic writing, but they still pop up, and when they do, they usually drag along extra words, as in the following examples:

These findings also have applicability to clinical practice.

Problems of less difficulty are always at the beginning of the list.

Tavish and McDonald's conclusions of greatest importance are summarized next.

Simplifying the adjectives and trimming unnecessary words enhances readability:

The findings also apply to clinical practice.

Less difficult problems always are at the beginning of the list.

Tavish and McDonald's most important conclusions are summarized next.

Appropriate Nominalization

Eliminating awkward nominalizations can make writing clearer and more concise, but not every nominalization creates a problem. A nominalization can enhance cohesion among sentences by linking the subject of a sentence to a preceding sentence, often with a relative pronoun such as "this," "these," or "those":

These observations support the hypothesis.

The deviation was not great enough to compromise reliability.

Some nominalizations save words and rescue sentences from awkwardness. Common nominalizations such as "analysis," "recovery," "performance," and "classification" serve important purposes in academic and technical writing and are appropriate provided they do not drag along excess lexical baggage. Nominals that function as the head of a noun phrase often yield simple and easy-to-comprehend sentences. Sentences with a lead-in nominal read more smoothly than sentences in which the nominal is replaced by a verb:

Lead-in nominal: *Participants' performance in the pretest determined their group assignments.*

Nominal replaced by a verb: *How well participants performed in the pretest determined their group assignments.*

Gerunds (nouns formed from verbs by adding *-ing*, as in "assigning," "measuring," and "adding") are nominalizations of a sort. Because a gerund functions as a noun, it may occupy the same sentence positions (e.g., subject, direct object, object of a preposition) as true nouns. Although gerunds are nominals, they usually do not add to wordiness. When used wisely, they can eliminate verbal clutter, as in

Swallowing requires the collaboration of many muscle groups. (Gerund as subject.)

for

When a person swallows the collaboration of many muscle groups is required.

Effective meditation requires slow and rhythmic breathing. (Gerund as direct object.)

for

Effective meditation requires that participants breathe slowly and rhythmically.

Infinitives often are interchangeable with gerunds. Infinitives may function as sentence subjects, as in

To write well is not easy.

or as direct objects, as in

I like to write.

Like gerunds, infinitives often provide an efficient way to express an idea:

Writing well is not easy.—To write well is not easy.

I like writing.—I like to write.

How do we choose? Often the rhythm of the sentence will tell you. An infinitive usually gives greater emphasis than does a gerund. "To write" (infinitive) in these examples improves sentence rhythm and highlights the act of writing better than does "writing" (gerund).

Watch for nominals in your writing. When you nominalize, consider whether the nominalization serves a useful purpose. If it does not, rewrite the sentence in a simpler, more direct way. But you need not prune out every nominalization. Keep those that link sentences or contribute to conciseness and clarity. Eradicate those that add useless words and weigh down your sentences.

Conjunctions and Modifiers as Sources of Clutter

When you have cleaned up sentence beginnings, have replaced weak verbs with strong verbs, and have selectively pruned nominalizations, turn your attention to conjunctions and modifiers—common sources of lexical excess.

Smothered Conjunctions

Conjunctions are among the most common and hardest-working English words. These small but mighty words play an important part in creating coherence in a text by showing relationships among ideas. Conjunctions link clauses in such sentences as

> *Andrew left the party early because his ex-wife showed up with her handsome new boyfriend in his bright red Maserati Granturismo convertible.*

If hard-working conjunctions are replaced by heavy-handed phrases such as "in the event that," "in spite of the fact that," and "for the reason that," coherence plummets, and readers' workload escalates. The conjunctions "if" and "although" frequently fall victim to such lexical gussying up, as in

> *In the event that (If) at least eight of ten judges did not agree on the classification of an item, the item was discarded.*

> *The order of conditions was counterbalanced in spite of the fact that (although) we did not expect an order effect.*

Overweight phrases substituting for "because" are especially common in scientific and academic writing:

> *Nonparametric statistics were calculated, based on the fact that (because) the data were not normally distributed.*

> *Three participants were dismissed as a consequence of (because of) their failure to pass the screening test.*

The last example shows how phrases such as "as a consequence of" add to wordiness by provoking nominalization of trailing verbs—in this example, "failure to pass" for "did not pass." Getting rid of the wordy lead-in phrase permits replacement of the nominal with a strong verb and produces a streamlined sentence:

> *Three participants were dismissed because they did not pass the screening test.*

Smothered Adverbs

Some writers avoid adverbs, perhaps because they are uncertain about when to use them and how to spell them. Writers who are uncertain about adverbs are uncertain with reason. Most adverbs end in *-ly* (e.g., slowly, carefully, bravely, legibly), but some do not (e.g., often, now, soon, later, always). To complicate matters more ("more" is an adverb), some adjectives end in *-ly* (e.g., friendly, lonely, costly, daily).

Adverbs may add color to plain verbs, but when a capable stand-alone adverb is replaced by an adverbial phrase, clutter follows. Some writers, either from habit or from a desire to dress their prose in fancy clothes, insert an adverbial phrase in which an adjective and a noun stand in for the adverb, as in

> *The data were collected in a careful way.*

which can be written in a more concise way (written more concisely) as

> *The data were carefully collected.*

Two adverbial phrases weigh down the following sentence:

On all occasions write in a concise manner.

which condenses to

Always write concisely.

Adverbs relating actions to time (e.g., then, now, soon, later, today, promptly) are common victims of adverbial glut. Instead of "now," sentences are burdened with "at the present time," "at this point in time," "as of the present," or similarly wordy substitutes. Instead of "soon," we see "in the near future," or "at an early date." Instead of "later," we see "at a future time":

The reasons for the discrepancy in results cannot at this time be determined.

which is better written as

The reasons for the discrepancy in results cannot now be determined.

(The last example would be better without "now." "Now" is implied by the present tense of the verb.)

Here is another example of adverbial overkill relating to time:

At this point in time there is no conclusive link between smoking and hypertension.

The word "present" implies time. Getting rid of the adverbial phrase saves two words:

At present there is no conclusive link between smoking and hypertension.

Better yet, get rid of "at present" and save two more words. "Is" implies now:

There is no conclusive link between smoking and hypertension.

Adverbs functioning as qualifiers (e.g., apparently, perhaps, partly, completely) are not immune to padding, as in

Instead of:
It would appear that Buckminster and Fuller anticipated the demise of their model.

Use:
Buckminster and Fuller apparently anticipated the demise of their model.

Instead of:
It may be that the model does not provide a complete account of the process.

Use:
Perhaps the model does not provide a complete account of the process.

But while we're at it, let's also get rid of the nominalization in the last example:

Perhaps the model does not completely explain the process.

Smothered Adjectives

Adjectives, like adverbs, sometimes fall victim to lexical gussying-up. Adjectives expressing quantity, such as "much," "few," "many," and "must" often are victims. "Much" is replaced by "a considerable amount of." "Few" is replaced by "a small number of." "Many" is replaced by "a large number of." "Most" is replaced by "a majority of":

This phenomenon has been described in a large number of (many) published articles.

A majority of the (Most) medications currently on the market are ineffective as treatments for dementia.

A sentence with a heavy-handed adjectival phrase often can be cleaned up by substituting a participle for the phrase. A participle is a word created by adding *-ing* or *-ed* to a verb. Participles may function as adjectives to modify nouns or pronouns (e.g., a flying bird, a falling rock, a cracked dish, a folded paper):

Instead of:

Findings that are related to this hypothesis are discussed next.

Use:

Findings related to this hypothesis are discussed next.

Instead of:

Unfortunately we cannot recover the data that are missing.

Use:

Unfortunately we cannot recover the missing data.

Unnecessary Redundancy as a Source of Clutter

All comprehensible written material is redundant. Writers use redundancy to ease readers' workload, to unify elements of text, and to emphasize important information. Writers create redundancy by repeating words, by establishing connections with synonyms or pronoun referents, and by paraphrasing previously mentioned elements of a text.

The boldface words in the next example connect elements in the second sentence to elements in the first by repeating information from the first sentence and by using a pronoun to refer to a previous referent:

*Ten judges rated the cohesiveness of the narratives. Each **judge** had previously received four hours of training to prepare **them** for rating the narratives.*

The next example shows how paraphrase adds redundancy and enhances readability:

Efficient readers use cohesive devices as markers indicating what is important and to what they should pay attention as they read.

In this example, the phrase "to what they should pay attention" paraphrases "what is important" to emphasize the idea that cohesive devices help to highlight important information in a text. This example also shows how parallel structure can unify elements of text. Parallel structure denotes the use of repeated word patterns to show that ideas are related and of equivalent importance. Some textual redundancy is indispensable. It provides readers with cues regarding the relationships of elements in a text. Without redundancy, texts become disjointed and difficult or impossible to comprehend.

But texts may be too redundant. Unnecessary redundancy interferes with comprehension because readers must read around redundant words to make sense of overly redundant texts. Unnecessary redundancy tarnishes much scientific and scholarly writing. It is a prominent contributor to the awkward, tedious prose that some consider a hallmark of the genre.[1]

Empty Modifiers

Some writers use adjectives and adverbs as verbal throat clearings ("ahem" words), used more from habit than by intent. These empty modifiers (in bold below) do little more than take up space and delay getting to the point:

> Phrenology **generally** fell into disrepute by the end of the 19th century.

> Though your manuscript adds nothing new, it is **basically** well written.

> This **particular** medication is not appropriate for juveniles.

Redundant Modifiers

Redundant modifiers—modifiers that convey the same information as the word(s) they modify—are a common source of excess redundancy in science writing:

> Systematic study of the relationship between brain structures and behavior first began in the 18th century.

"Began" is sufficient. "First began" is overkill. You would not write "second began" or "third began," so do not write "first began."

Here is a redundancy that often pops up in scientific writing as well as in the popular press and in radio and television broadcasts:

> The literature search yielded a grand total of 492 citations.

> A grand total of 12 people were killed by the tornado.

"Grand total" is senseless. If totals may be grand, may they not also be modest, piddling, or puny? Cutting out "grand" does not, however, save the sentence:

> The literature search yielded a total of 492 citations.

> A total of 12 people were killed by the tornado.

Redemption comes only when "a total of" is gone:

> The literature search yielded 492 citations.

> Twelve people were killed by the tornado.

We suspect that "a total of" was first written by someone who knew he or she should not begin a sentence with a numeral but wanted to duck spelling it out. Sentences that begin with "a total of" are at least 10 times as frequent as sentences in which "a total of" appears later. Don't clutter your writing with this redundancy. If the sentence begins with a number, spell out the number. If you are

---

[1]Students in some writing classes have been taught not to repeat a noun, verb, adjective, or adverb within a certain number of sentences because such repetition was believed to contribute to monotonous prose. A writer constrained by such a rule might write in successive sentences that a character frowned, then grimaced, then scowled, and eventually glowered. Though perhaps acceptable in novels, short stories, poetry, and other works of creative fiction, such verbal gymnastics have no place in technical writing.

reluctant to do that, rewrite the sentence to move the number back, as we have done in the next example:

The tornado killed 12 people.

Leave "a total of" to radio and television. There it is endemic, and there is no cure.

Redundant Categories

Many words imply the names of their category. "Red" denotes color. "Large" denotes size. "Heavy" denotes weight. Writing both the word and the name of its category is overkill:

The tokens were large or small in size and red or blue in color.

Participants were recruited in the month of May.

Brain tissue is soft in consistency and pink in color.

Getting rid of redundant category names also gets rid of connecting words such as "in," "the," and "of":

The tokens were large or small and red or blue.

Participants were recruited in May.

Brain tissue is soft and pink.

A noun separated from a modifier by a preposition (usually "in" or "of") warns of unnecessary redundancy. Watch for such combinations as you edit, and when you find one, repair it, unless they add emphasis or improve the rhythm of the sentence.

Empty or redundant modifiers can be stealthy, because being habitual, they creep undetected into what we write as we are preoccupied with getting our thoughts down on paper. No matter. They are easier to spot when you copy edit, so get rid of them then.

Passive Voice as a Source of Clutter

Indiscriminate use of passive voice is an important contributor to the overblown style that some consider a hallmark of academic writing. For readers who have forgotten the difference between active voice and passive voice, here is a short tutorial.

In active sentences, the subject (the agent, or doer of the action) precedes the verb, and the recipient of the action (the object) follows the verb, as in

Marie (agent) opened (verb) the letter (recipient).

The editor (agent) rejected (verb) the manuscript (recipient).

In passive sentences, the recipient of the action precedes the verb, and the agent follows the verb, as in

The letter (recipient) was opened (verb) by Marie (agent).

The manuscript (recipient) was rejected (verb) by the editor (agent).

Passive sentences usually require more words than active sentences—a preposition (usually "by") to link the verb to the agent, and an auxiliary verb (usually "is," "are," "was," or "were") to convert the main verb into passive form.

Passive sentences are infrequent in everyday English texts but are common in scientific and academic writing. About 10% of sentences in scientific and academic articles are passive, versus about 4% in works of fiction (Quirk, Greenbaum, Leech, & Svartvik, 1985; Xiao, McEnery, & Qian, 2006).

Passive voice has been a favorite target of style manuals and writing gurus for many years. Passive voice got much of its bad reputation from generations of bureaucrats, politicians, and public officials who used passive voice to impress, confuse, or duck responsibility:

The documents were destroyed under the terms of XYZ corporation's policies on retention of records.

Misleading information regarding profitability was provided in XYZ corporation's annual report.

Discrepancies in the report were found but were not considered serious.

Active voice encourages the writer to name the person or group who did whatever was done:

J. Smith and P. Doe destroyed the records under the terms of XYZ corporation's policies on retention of records.

The XYZ corporation board of directors provided misleading information regarding profitability in the corporation's annual report.

The company auditor found discrepancies in the report but did not consider them serious.

Favoring active voice makes good sense, because sentences in active voice are more direct and more efficient than are sentences in passive voice. "Marie opened the letter" is two words shorter than "The letter was opened by Marie." "The editor rejected the manuscript" is two words shorter than "The manuscript was rejected by the editor." In addition to saving words, active sentences are more vigorous than passive sentences because the agent occupies the driver's seat:

"A did something to B" is more lively than "Something was done to B by A."

The simplest way to make a passive sentence into an active sentence is to make the agent of the action the subject and the recipient of the action the object of the verb. The agent in a passive sentence usually is a noun that follows the word "by," as in

The kazoo band was booed by the audience.

Converting the sentence to active voice yields

The audience booed the kazoo band.

wherein the positions of the agent and the recipient are transposed.

Another way to change a passive sentence into an active sentence is to change the verb. Changing the verb is a good way to create an active sentence that retains the word order of the passive sentence:

Many trees were killed by the drought. (passive)

Converting the sentence to active voice by changing the verb yields

Many trees died because of the drought. (active)

As you edit, be especially watchful for nominalizations that occupy the sentence subject position, because such nominalizations typically introduce passive sentences with undefined agents:

Measurement of protein levels was accomplished by application of the XYZ procedure, which enabled specification of the underlying metabolic processes.

Changing nominals to verbs and rewriting sentences in active voice makes for simpler, clearer sentences. The revised sentences will be about one third shorter than the nominalized sentences:

We measured protein levels with the XYZ procedure to specify the underlying metabolic processes.

Here are a few more example sentences with lead-in nominalizations:

The specification of criterion levels was accomplished utilizing measurements of great precision.

Our reliance on measures of borderline precision resulted in a reduction of the accuracy and reliability of our results.

Determination of the magnitude of treatment effects was accomplished utilizing the Yates procedure.

First get rid of the nominalizations:

Precise measures were used to specify criterion levels.

The inaccurate and unreliable results were caused by our imprecise measures.

The magnitude of treatment effects was measured utilizing the Yates procedure.

Then rewrite in active voice:

We specified criterion levels with precise measures.

Our imprecise measures caused inaccurate and unreliable results.

We measured treatment effects with the Yates procedure.

Passive voice does, however, have its uses. If it did not, it would have disappeared by now. Passive voice is appropriate when the recipient of an action rather than the agent is the focus of a sentence. In a story about a politician named Smith, a reporter might write this passive sentence:

Smith was accused by the district attorney of converting campaign funds to his personal use.

If the story were about Smith's trial on the charge, the reporter might write an active sentence:

The district attorney accused Smith of converting campaign funds to his personal use.

Passive sentences often enhance the continuity of text. The author of an article about telemarketing calls might write

The Federal Trade Commission is considering regulations that would protect consumers from unwanted telemarketing calls. Telemarketing calls were called "unwarranted invasions of privacy" by the National Consumers Federation.

By placing telemarketing calls at the beginning of the second sentence, the passive second sentence tells the reader that the topic is telemarketing calls. An active sentence in its place, as in the following example, leaves the reader wondering if the focus of the article has changed from telemarketing calls to the National Consumers Federation:

> *The Federal Trade Commission is considering regulations that would protect consumers from unwanted telemarketing calls. The National Consumers Federation has labeled telemarketing calls "unwarranted invasions of privacy."*

When the agent of an action is obvious, unknown, or unimportant, a passive sentence is a good choice:

> *Big Sky Airways' flight schedule was changed on June 1.*

> *The* Journal of Questionable Research *is published twice a year.*

> *The Little Joy hummingbird feeder is made of durable plastic.*

The preceding three sentences differ from the other examples because they do not specify an agent. Such sentences are known as truncated passives, partial passives, or agentless passives. Truncated passives are from 10 to 20 times more frequent than are full passives in English printed materials (Xiao et al., 2006). Full passives rarely occur in spoken English. Less than 5% of utterances in everyday spoken English are truncated passives (Bresnan, Dingare, & Manning, 2001).

In contrast to the preferences of everyday English speakers and writers, passive sentences have long been a favorite of writers of scientific and technical

works because they are thought to signify unbiased reporting. Consider the following passage, which might appear in the introduction to a research article written in the style favored by some writers of scientific articles:

> *Sleep disturbances often are experienced by people with chronic obstructive pulmonary disease (COPD). Sleep disturbances are experienced by people with COPD when night-time blood oxygen levels fall enough to cause discomfort. The abnormally low night-time blood oxygen levels are believed to be a result of compromised pulmonary function. (50 words)*

The glut of passive sentences in the preceding passage makes for tedious reading. Replacing passive sentences with active sentences and eliminating unneeded redundancy improves continuity, enhances readability, and gets rid of 12 words of clutter:

> *People with chronic obstructive pulmonary disease (COPD) often have sleep disturbances, which appear when night-time blood oxygen levels fall enough to cause discomfort. Compromised pulmonary function causes blood oxygen levels to fall, creates discomfort, and disrupts sleep. (38 words)*

Passive sentences do, however, have a legitimate place in technical and scientific writing. In scientific and technical writing (as in other kinds of writing), full passives allow the writer to focus discourse—if the agent is not the focus, passives allow the writer to remove it from the subject position. For example, in the introduction of an article on models of memory, an author might write the following first sentence:

The dual-trace model of memory was first described by Bell, Book, and Candle (1954).

which implies that the topic is the dual-trace model of memory. Making the sentence an active sentence, as in

Bell, Book, and Candle (1954) first described the dual-trace model of memory.

suggests that the topic is Bell, Book, and Candle.

Truncated passives are traditional in descriptions of experimental procedures, wherein what happened is more important than who did it:

Transcripts were typed into a computer file. Clause and sentence boundaries were identified and markers were inserted to demarcate them. Clause and sentence boundaries were identified using the Silverman and Sorfino procedure.

Writing such material in active voice requires tedious repetition of the person who performed the actions and changes the focus from the procedure to the person, which is not what procedures are about:

The experimenter typed the transcripts into a computer file. Then he identified clause and sentence boundaries and inserted markers to demarcate them. The experimenter identified clause and sentence boundaries using the Silverman and Sorfino procedure.

Passive sentences are useful in descriptions of procedures, including data acqui-

sition and analysis of results. The method and results sections of research articles may make liberal use of passives without compromising style or readability, although long strings of passives, like long strings of any sentence form, make text tedious and boring. Plan to bias your writing style toward passive sentences in the method and results sections, but bias it toward active sentences in the other sections of a research article. (See Chapter 3, The Method, and Chapter 4, The Results, for more on passive sentences in research articles.)

Using Ellipsis to Reduce Clutter

Ellipsis offers a clever way to cut unnecessary words. Ellipsis is grammarian lingo for deliberate omission of words that are obvious from context. Ellipsis reduces sentence length without sacrificing clarity or meaning. Consider the following paragraph:

Ellipsis can reduce sentence length without sacrificing sentence clarity or sentence meaning. Repeated words, redundant words, and contextually implied words may safely be deleted. Repeated words, redundant words, and contextually implied words may, however, be retained if they emphasize one or more ideas in a sentence.

This paragraph is weighed down with unneeded words. Deleting them (ellipsing them?) enhances readability. (We could have written, . . . enhances the paragraph's readability. Why didn't we?)

Ellipsis can reduce sentence length without sacrificing clarity or meaning. Repeated, redundant, and contextually implied words may safely be deleted unless they emphasize one or more ideas in a sentence.

The most obvious candidates for ellipsis are repeated words, as in

Five word lists contained familiar words, and five word lists contained unfamiliar words.

Ellipsis improves the sentence:

Five word lists contained familiar words, and five contained unfamiliar words.

Words implied by context are harder to spot but often are better deleted, as in

The data were reliable though they were incomplete.

in which the referent for "incomplete" is clear without "they were." Ellipsis improves the sentence:

The data were reliable, though incomplete.

Experienced writers routinely use ellipsis—usually without thinking about it. Inexperienced writers often fail to recognize opportunities for ellipsis. Writers of research articles may neglect ellipsis because they fail to give readers credit for grasping what is implied but unsaid. They may write redundant, wordy sentences because they feel compelled to take specificity to a level at which there is no possibility that any reader will misunderstand. Or they may wish to make lackluster ideas appear impressive.

Using Punctuation to Eliminate Clutter

Punctuation can be another useful tool for eliminating unneeded words. A colon or a dash may replace lead-in words or phrases that introduce lists:

Instead of:

To pass the screening test, participants had to correctly name line drawings of five common objects. The drawings were pencil, fork, key, comb, and cup.

Use:

To pass the screening test, participants had to correctly name line drawings of five common objects: pencil, fork, key, comb, and cup.

Instead of:

Several characteristics affect the comprehensibility of sentences. The characteristics are syntax, length, phonologic complexity, and word familiarity.

Use:

Several characteristics affect the comprehensibility of sentences— syntax, length, phonologic complexity, and word familiarity.

A dash may replace words that introduce comments or explanations:

Regional populations, which are rounded to the nearest hundred thousand, are shown in Table 1.

Regional populations—rounded to the nearest hundred thousand—are shown in Table 1.

Parentheses also may be used to set off comments or explanations and eliminate lead-in phrases:

Regional populations (rounded to the nearest hundred thousand) are shown in Table 1.

Parentheses are less obtrusive than dashes, and sentences with parentheses usually read more smoothly than sentences with dashes. When you have a choice, favor parentheses.

Modifiers

If clutter is gone and the words are well chosen but a sentence still does not say exactly what you intend, scrutinize the modifiers. Misplaced modifiers are a common cause of vague, ambiguous, or misleading sentence meaning.

Accurate placement of modifiers (words, phrases, or clauses) is an important source of clarity in texts. A modifier is misplaced if readers cannot quickly connect it to the word it modifies (its referent). At best, sentences with misplaced modifiers are awkward. At worst, they are confusing or misleading. Sometimes they are unintentionally humorous:

We have a nursery for those who have children and don't know it.

Cook vegetables and fruit that cannot be peeled during bouts of diarrhea.

Three tests were chosen by the authors; they were short and simple.

Put modifiers near the word(s) they modify. Readers automatically try to link a modifier to the nearest word(s) it could modify. If too many words intervene between a modifier and its referent, readers must work to make the connection between the modifier and its referent, and may make the wrong connection.

Limiting Modifiers

Limiting modifiers (modifiers such as "only," "almost," "nearly," "scarcely," "exactly," "hardly," "just," and "simply" that restrict or limit the meaning of their referents) are especially sensitive to placement. Readers expect a limiting modifier to modify the idea that immediately follows it, so place most limiting modifiers just before their referents. Changing the location of a limiting modifier may have strong effects on the meaning of a sentence:

Only the treated group passed the test. (Other groups did not pass the test.)

The treated group only passed the test. (Ambiguous. Other groups did not pass or the treated group nearly failed the test.)

The treated group passed only the test. (The treated group did not pass anything else.)

The treated group passed the only test. (Only one test was given, and the treated group passed it.)

Squinting Modifiers

Sometimes the placement of a modifier creates ambiguity about which of two (or sometimes more than two) ideas it modifies.

Such ambiguously placed modifiers are called *squinting modifiers*. Here is an example of a squinting modifier:

> *Participants who were instructed* **carefully** *monitored the visual display.*

Two close-by potential referents for "carefully" create ambiguity. Was the instruction done with care, or did the participants monitor with care? Relocation of the adverb resolves the ambiguity:

> *Participants who were carefully instructed monitored the visual display.* (Instruction was done with care.)

> *Participants who were instructed monitored carefully the visual display.* (Participants monitored with care.)

> *Participants who were instructed monitored the visual display carefully.* (Participants monitored with care.)

Dangling Modifiers

A dangling modifier is a word, phrase, or clause that seems to modify the wrong word(s) or does not logically modify any word or words in a sentence. We call them *orphan modifiers*. Dangling modifiers usually are clauses or phrases that begin a sentence and contain verb forms but do not identify a sentence subject.

Dangling modifiers usually introduce otherwise complete sentences, as in the following example:

> *Testing at the single-word level, no abnormal performance was found.*

Repair this by giving the dangling modifier a subject (in this example, "participants" is the subject):

> *When we tested participants at the single-word level, we found no abnormal performance.*

Sometimes dangling modifiers are tacked on to the end of a sentence:

> *The board found several flaws in design, canceling the project.*

Fix this by combining the dangling phrase or clause and the main clause into a single sentence:

> *The board found several flaws in design and canceled the project.*

Dangling modifiers often introduce passive sentences:

> *After analyzing the data, no treatment effect was found.*

Fix this by changing the subject of the main clause to a word the dangling modifier describes:

> *After I analyzed the data I found no treatment effect.*

Pronouns

Misplaced pronouns (pronouns that do not unambiguously refer to a single nearby referent) always increase readers' workload and often confuse or mislead them. An unclear pronoun reference usually has one of three causes.

There is more than one possible referent for the pronoun, as in

> *Because the patient's brain tumor was so difficult to reach, the surgeon operated on his knees.*

The referent is too far away from the pronoun, as in

Teachers often have commented on poor readers' difficulty pronouncing phonologically complex words and separating words into syllables— difficulties for which causes have not been identified. They rely on intuition and experience as guides.

The referent is implied but not named:

Jones defended his theory in 1980, but it was not published.

Place pronouns close enough to their referents to prevent ambiguity. Be especially careful in placing dependent clauses beginning with "that," "which," or "who." Put them immediately after their referents. If you intend this,

Each person who agreed to participate was interviewed by an intern.

Do not write this:

Each person was interviewed by an intern who agreed to participate.

Do not identify an otherwise ambiguous referent parenthetically, as in

Jones, in discussing Smith's model, asserted that he (Smith) had not considered the full range of possible outcomes.

Instead, revise the sentence to clarify the identity of the referent by placing the pronoun near its referent:

Jones asserted that Smith, in his model, had not considered the full range of possible outcomes.

Use relative pronouns such as "this," "that," "which," and "it" carefully when the pronoun refers to an idea or concept described in the preceding text. Be sure that the connection between the words introduced by the relative pronoun and the content of the preceding text will be obvious to readers:

Metacognition denotes the ability to think about one's cognitive processes and to be aware of one's mental activities during activities such as problem solving, listening, and reading. This is a major determinant of one's competence for independent living in daily life.

In this example, the referent for "this" is ambiguous because it relates to the idea of the preceding statement rather than to specific words in the statement. Because readers expect pronouns to refer to specific elements of adjacent text, they will first search the text for nouns that might substitute for the pronoun, beginning with those nearest the pronoun—in this example, reading, listening, problem solving, cognitive processes, ability, metacognition—none of which are satisfactory because the referent is an idea, not a word. Spelling out the referent resolves the ambiguity:

Metacognition denotes the ability to think about one's cognitive processes and to be aware of one's mental activities during activities such as problem solving, listening, and reading. The ability to think about one's cognitive processes is a major determinant of one's competence for independent living in daily life.

Implied ideas are ambiguous referents for pronouns. An idea may be implied by a word or a phrase but cannot serve as a referent for a pronoun:

> *The effects of treatment were evaluated with a t-test, but it was not significant.*

We see statements such as this in many manuscripts and always mark them for revision. Statistical tests are not significant in themselves, but only indicate whether trends or relationships in the data are statistically significant. To resolve the ambiguity, provide the implied referent—in this case, the relationships extracted from the data:

> *The effects of treatment were evaluated with a t-test, but the difference between the treatment group and the control group was not significant.*

Here is another example of an implied idea as a pronoun referent:

> *The durations of eye fixations in reading vary widely. Fixations on function words are brief, fixations on unusual words and words at the ends of sentences are longer. This is why their reading rate for technical text is slower than their rate for nontechnical text.*

In this example, the pronoun "their" refers not to words or ideas mentioned in the preceding sentences, but to readers whose presence is only implied. Providing the implied referent resolves the ambiguity:

> *The durations of eye fixations in reading vary widely. Fixations on function words are brief; fixations on unusual words and words at the ends of sentences are longer. This is why a reader's reading rate for technical*

> *text is slower than their rate for nontechnical text.*

Do not use a pronoun to refer to an adjective or a possessive noun. Although an adjective or a possessive noun may imply a noun, an implied noun cannot serve as a referent for a pronoun:

> *In Smith's discussion, he claimed support for his hypothesis.*

In this example, "Smith's" functions as a possessive adjective modifying "discussion." Using it as the referent for "he" creates an awkward sentence, although most readers may figure out that the writer intends that "he" refers to "Smith." To improve the sentence, substitute the referent for the pronoun:

> *In Smith's discussion, Smith claimed support for his hypothesis.*

Better yet, rewrite it without the introductory phrase:

> *Smith claimed support for his hypothesis in his discussion.*

or

> *In his discussion, Smith claimed support for his hypothesis.*

The pronoun "it" has three common uses: as a personal pronoun (e.g., Each story was recorded on audiotape. Then it was transcribed by a skilled typist.), as an idiomatic expression (e.g., It is cold.), and to postpone the subject of a sentence (e.g., It is poor form to use "impact" as a verb.). Do not mix the uses within a sentence:

> *It is poor form to use impact as a verb, because it is a noun.*

To repair such sentences, replace an "it" with its referent:

> *It is poor form to use impact as a verb, because impact is a noun.*

Or, when an introductory phrase beginning with "it" begins a sentence, rewrite the sentence without the introductory phrase:

> *Impact is a noun; do not use it as a verb.*

Getting rid of an introductory phrase often gives a sentence more punch, as it does here. (We believe the referent for "it" in this assertion is clear.)

Infinitives: To Split or Not to Split

For 150 years, student writers have been warned not to split infinitives. That prohibition now has been tossed in the dustbin, save for a few remaining fusspots who believe that splitting an infinitive may be done only in private with the doors locked and the curtains closed.

Infinitives in English typically consist of the marker "to" plus the uninflected form of a verb, as in

> *To sleep, perchance to dream.*

> *To err is human, to forgive is divine.*

> *Phyllis decided to drive around the parking lot while waiting for a parking space for her new Lamborghini.*

> *Tell the contractor to make the repairs.*

A split infinitive is created when a word or phrase (usually an adverb or an adverbial phrase) is placed between the word "to" and the verb, as in

> *To inevitably sleep, to perchance dream.*

> *To unintentionally err is human, to intentionally forgive is divine.*

> *Phyllis decided to slowly drive around the parking lot while waiting for a parking space for her new Lamborghini.*

> *Tell the contractor to quickly and completely make the repairs.*

Split infinitives attracted little notice until the 19th century, when their increasing frequency in the English spoken by educated and erudite Britons and in published works of the time drew the attention of grammarians and language purists, including one Henry Alford, who condemned split infinitives in a then well-known manual of idiom called *A Plea for the Queen's English*, published in 1863. During the next several decades, grammarians and language purists hopped on the no-split bandwagon, and split infinitives largely disappeared from the speech of educated Britons and from literary works in England and the United States. (Split infinitives have never been common in everyday conversational English.)

Reaction to the no-split movement was not long in coming. By the early 20th century grammarians, and writers began to stand up for splitting:

> *The split infinitive has taken such hold upon the consciences of journalists that, instead of warning the novice against splitting his infinitives, we must warn him against the curious superstition that the splitting or not splitting makes the difference between a good and a bad writer* (Fowler & Fowler, 1908, p. 319)

Writers in science and academia ought to be prudent with infinitive splitting to avoid offending the remaining purists who frown on the practice. Although splitting infinitives is now considered acceptable, most style manuals recommend that they not be split unless the split version is clearer, easier to read, and easier to understand than the nonsplit version.

Placing infinitive-splitting adverbs in front of or behind infinitives is the most common way to avoid splitting them. Splitting the infinitive in this sentence makes for awkwardness:

To effortlessly write requires great effort.

Putting the adverb after the infinitive improves rhythm and readability:

To write effortlessly requires great effort.

But putting the adverb before the infinitive would be a mistake:

Effortlessly to write requires great effort.

Sometimes changing the location of an adverb relative to an infinitive changes a sentence's meaning. Consider the following sentence in which an adverb splits the infinitive:

Experienced writers remember to clearly define technical terms.

"Clearly" unambiguously modifies "define" in this sentence. Putting the adverb before the infinitive suggests that the remembering was clear:

Experienced writers remember clearly to define technical terms.

Putting the adverb after the infinitive suggests that experienced writers define only obviously technical terms:

Experienced writers remember to define clearly technical terms.

Splitting infinitives with negations is frowned upon by many who are otherwise tolerant of split infinitives:

Sometimes it is wise to not follow a rule.

I hereby resolve to never split an infinitive.

Style manuals usually caution against such split-infinitive constructions and recommend that writers refrain from splitting infinitives that are modified by negations, and that the proper place for the negation is before the infinitive:

Sometimes it is wise not to follow a rule.

I hereby resolve never to split an infinitive.

Be cautious about splitting infinitives in which several adverbs or a long adverbial phrase intervene between "to" and the verb, as in

We intend to carefully, systematically, and completely scrutinize the results to ensure their accuracy.

Moving the adverbs to keep the infinitive unsplit improves readability:

We intend to scrutinize the results carefully, systematically, and completely to ensure their accuracy.

One way to avoid the split-infinitive issue is to rewrite a sentence to eliminate the infinitive altogether. The sentence,

Experienced writers remember to clearly define technical terms.

may be rewritten as

Experienced writers clearly define technical terms.

The sentence,

To effortlessly write requires great effort.

may be rewritten as

Effortless writing requires great effort.

Sometimes rewriting to remove an infinitive improves a sentence, as in "Effortless writing requires great effort," but rewriting sometimes produces awkward, difficult-to-read sentences, as in the following example, wherein the first sentence reads smoothly and unambiguously despite the presence of an infinitive:

The premier promised the insurgents amnesty to end the war.

Rewriting this sentence without an infinitive creates an awkward sentence in which a wordy phrase replaces a more efficient infinitive:

The premier promised the insurgents amnesty if they would end the war.

The rewriting option is always available but may not always be worth the effort, especially if rewriting lessens the quality of a sentence. With infinitives, as with other constructions, the objective is to make sentences simple, direct, unambiguous, and easy for the reader to understand. If rewriting a sentence to get rid of an infinitive adds clutter, keep the infinitive.

Adverbs in Compound Verbs: To Split or Not to Split

A compound verb (sometimes called a verb phrase) consists of an auxiliary verb plus a main verb. Most English auxiliary verbs can form compound verbs but cannot stand alone as main verbs. The exceptions are the words "be," "have," and "do," and their various forms, which can function either as auxiliaries or as main verbs. The remaining auxiliary verbs (can/could, may/might, must/ought, shall/should, and will/would) can function only as auxiliaries. Here are four sentences with compound verbs:

The participants in this study were selected from elementary schools in Chagrin Falls, Idaho.

I learned today that the editor had rejected my manuscript 3 weeks ago.

Deviating from these procedures will compromise interpretation of the results.

None of these medications are thought to be without risk.

Sometimes writers choose to qualify a main verb or add color with an adverb, as in the following sentences:

The participants in this study were randomly selected from elementary schools in Chagrin Falls, Idaho.

I learned today that the editor had irrevocably rejected my manuscript 3 weeks ago.

Deviating from these procedures will seriously compromise interpretation of the results.

None of these medications are currently thought to be without risk.

Most writers paid scant attention to where to put adverbs modifying compound verbs until the 1970s, when newspaper journalists were told that it was against the rules to put an adverb between an auxiliary verb and a main verb, as in, "were randomly selected," "had irrevocably rejected," or "will seriously compromise." They were told that adverbs typically should precede auxiliary verbs, as in "randomly were selected," but sometimes could follow the main verb as in "had rejected irrevocably."

The origin of this stricture against splitting compound verbs is unknown, but it may reflect extension of the no-split rule from infinitives to compound verbs. The do-not-split rule for compound verbs was short-lived, perhaps because it caused many awkward sentences. Placing adverbs within compound verbs usually does not cause problems for readers, as in

Smith and Jones have carefully outlined the basic concepts in their model.

in which splitting the verb makes for a smoother, less awkward sentence than either unsplit version:

Smith and Jones carefully have outlined the basic concepts in their model.

Smith and Jones have outlined carefully the basic concepts in their model.

When a compound verb contains more than one auxiliary, most style manuals recommend that it follow the first auxiliary, as in the following sentence:

They would probably never have considered such an explanation.

Our advice—if you are inclined to put an adverb between the parts of a compound verb, go ahead. But do so only when the split version is clearer and creates a more rhythmic sentence than does the unsplit version.

Editing Verb Tense

Selecting verb tense in scientific papers can be a tricky business. Whether to write in past or present tense usually puzzles beginning writers and concerns experienced writers who sometimes find themselves unsure about whether to write in past tense or present tense. The following general principles should help.

When describing what has been done in the past, as in reviews of literature, past tense usually is appropriate:

Gannon, Gano, and Grandholm (1987) evaluated the reliability of the Michigan Assessment of Culinary Aptitude (MACA). They administered the MACA to a randomly selected sample of 100 cooking school applicants. They tested each applicant twice, with a one-week interval between tests.

Past tense is appropriate when you are writing about actions that began in the past and were completed in the past, as in the preceding example. When writing about conditions that are true in the present, present tense is appropriate. Thus,

Gannon, Gano, and Grandholm are the leading proponents of the "more is better" school of reliability analysis.

Sometimes past and present tense may be mixed into the same sentence:

Gannon, Gano, and Grandholm concluded that the MACA is not reliable enough to be used as a screening device when consistent selection criteria are desirable.

In this example, Gannon, Gano, and Grandholm came to their conclusion in the past, but what they concluded (we assume, with no evidence to the contrary) continues to the present.

The general principle: If you are writing about material that is true today, write in the present tense. Thus,

Einstein's work has a profound effect on how we think about the universe. When he concluded that time and space are related, most of his contemporaries were astonished.

Note that "concluded" (an action completed in the past) is in past tense, as is "astonished" (also an action—presumably—completed in the past). Some writers might write: "When he concluded that time and space were related . . . " to keep the tense of the adjacent verbs the same. That's probably acceptable, but "are" seems the better choice to us, because it signals the reader that the relationship still is considered true.

Procedures almost always are written in past tense:

Half of the participants were verbally praised on a semi-random schedule and the other half were given cash (25 cents) each time they detected a target.

Each participant's naming responses were tape-recorded. Their responses were scored for accuracy and completeness after the session ended.

Results generally are written in the past tense:

The performance of the two groups in the three conditions was evaluated with the Bgosh and Bgolly test for meaningful differences (Bgosh & Bgolly, 1995). The mean score for the control group was significantly less than the mean score for the experimental group in each condition.

Note that the second sentence in the foregoing example seems an exception to the principle of using present tense for material that continues to be true at present, if we assume that the mean scores remain significantly different even now. We would argue that it is not actually an exception, because the writer is reporting a statistical conclusion that was completed in the process of data analysis. Think of it this way:

The Bgosh and Bgolly test showed that the mean score for the control group was . . .

or

The mean score for the control group was found to be . . .

which makes past tense seem the better choice.

Present tense appears in the results sections of papers when the writer refers to tables and figures:

Table 1 shows the average scores for each participant.

Figure 1 shows the results, averaged across conditions.

The scores for each participant are provided in Appendix A.

Conclusions typically combine past tense and present tense. Past tense is used when referring to what happened during the planning and execution of the experiment and the analysis of results. Present tense typically is used when the writer makes statements relating to interpretation and implications of the results:

> *These results confirm certain cultural stereotypes—that female college students prefer decaffeinated coffee to caffeinated coffee, white wine to red wine, and soccer to American football, but that male college students prefer caffeinated coffee to decaffeinated coffee, beer to wine (either red or white), and world federation wrestling to all other sports. These findings were true even when the results were adjusted to account for differences in IQ scores between males and females. The female students' IQs were, on the average, 5 points greater than those of the male students.*

Note that the writer has put conclusions about results in present tense, but reverts to past tense when writing about data analysis procedures and results.

Word Choice and Precision

The difference between the right word and the almost right word is like the difference between lightning and a lightning bug. (Mark Twain)

The ideas that remain after you have cut out excess verbiage and have tightened sentence structure are the ideas that are likely to make it into the final draft. Now it's time to turn your editorial attention to the words and sentences that remain. Begin by searching out clichés, euphemisms, and inappropriately used technical lingo.

Clichés

Clichés are shopworn combinations of words that once expressed ideas in novel ways but have lost their sharpness because overuse has drained them of meaning. Clichés in everyday language are common:

> *It's music to my ears.*
>
> *The handwriting is on the wall.*
>
> *It's a dog eat dog world.*
>
> *There's no time like the present.*
>
> *Actions speak louder than words.*

Banalities such as these are common in everyday speech but uncommon in formal writing, wherein stylists frown upon them. Clichés that creep into formal writing are more subtle than everyday banalities. Clichés in formal writing, like clichés in informal speech and writing, are shopworn words and phrases that pop automatically into the writer's mind and from there onto the page.

Many clichés in scientific writing are adjective–noun combinations. Data are raw, alternatives are viable, facts are well-known, use is widespread, flaws are fatal, and change is sorely needed. Some clichés in scientific writing are stereotyped word pairs that are so overused that they are hackneyed and trite. They hammer home the meaning of a competent stand-alone word with another word that conveys the same meaning. "Each" is saddled with "and every." "Far" is encumbered with "and wide." "Over" is yoked to "and above."

The facts and figures are, by and large, over and above what is needed to compare and contrast the validity of the models.

We provide in the appendix a full and complete description of the procedures used to ensure the reliability of judges' ratings.

By these precautions we sought to eliminate each and every source of contamination.

Some clichés in scientific writing are trite phrases that interject several words where one or two would do. A conclusive finding is proved beyond a shadow of a doubt. An unlikely event cannot occur by any stretch of the imagination. A usual occurrence happens more often than not:

Contrary to popular opinion, for reasons too numerous to mention but needless to say by no stretch of the imagination can these results be construed as hard and fast confirmation of the theory.

Some clichés began as well-defined technical jargon, but lost their precision upon adoption into common English. Sometimes they find their way into scientific writing having nothing to do with the technical field from which the jargon comes. Recorders interface with amplifiers. Technicians input numbers into a database. Experimenters give feedback to participants. Faculty update their vitae.

But not all clichés are taboo. Some have retained at least some of their sharpness and, when used effectively, allow writers to communicate more effectively than if forced to detour around them. Sometimes a cliché is the most direct way of expressing a thought, and attempting to write around the cliché may lead to awkward and wordy text. To recommend that results be taken at face value communicates meaning beyond that easily obtained by words such as "believed" or "accepted."

Include clichés in your writing sparingly and with discretion. Shun them when they substitute for precise thought. Never use a cliché when you can say precisely the same thing with other words.

Euphemisms

Euphemisms are circumspect ways of expressing concepts that one has a reason for not expressing bluntly—usually to avoid offending another. We say "he passed away" or "he expired" instead of "he died." In social interactions, euphemisms provide an agreed-upon way of expressing potentially offensive content without upsetting others, but when overdone, euphemisms transcend courtesy and become affectations.

Euphemisms are common in diplomatic language, wherein they provide a country's representatives with a way of removing provocation from otherwise provocative statements. The diplomat who says, "We have reservations regarding the accuracy of the ambassador's assertions" is less likely to start a war than one who says, "We think the ambassador is lying."

Some euphemisms misrepresent reality. When a surgeon says, "The patient suffered an adverse outcome," we know that the patient either got worse or died ("bought the farm"). The politician who says, "We are in a period of negative economic growth," has chosen not to say, "We are in a recession." The military officer who says, "The mission was accompanied by significant collateral damage," has elected not to say, "We destroyed a lot of property and killed some innocent civilians."

Conventional euphemisms are not common in scientific and technical writing—perhaps because most readers of scientific and technical works are unlikely to be offended by bluntness. Not so for euphemisms that conceal or misrepresent reality. The writer who writes, "A trend toward significance was found" hopes readers will not notice that nothing was significant. The writer who characterizes results as "preliminary" and studies as "pilot" may be hoping that readers will not hold him or her to traditional standards for scientific merit.

Person-First Terminology

In the past, it was common in published works to see adjectives denoting groups with disabilities or adverse medical conditions converted to nouns and used to identify the groups and persons in the groups (e.g., epileptics, diabetics, schizophrenics, aphasics):

The group of aphasics comprised 10 Broca's aphasics, 10 Wernicke's aphasics, and 10 conduction aphasics.

These appellations largely disappeared during the 1970s, replaced by adjective–noun labels (e.g., epileptic adult, diabetic patients, schizophrenic person, aphasic individuals). In the 1980s, some groups began advocating person-first terminology when writers or speakers refer to persons or groups with disabilities or adverse medical conditions, apparently in the belief that referring to the person before referring to the disability avoids dehumanization of persons with disabilities. A "brain-injured adult" becomes an "adult who has a brain injury." "Diabetic patient" becomes "patient who has diabetes." "Obese adult" becomes "adult with obesity." (Or, taking the latter appellation further down a politically correct road, "adult with a weight issue.")

Some groups of disabled people reject person-first terminology because they believe that it devalues an important aspect of their identity and because it suggests that the disability and the person are separate entities. Many disability-rights activists in the United States consider person-first terminology euphemistic. Regardless of one's philosophical beliefs, person-first terminology contributes to wordiness, because it adds a preposition (e.g., person with aphasia, person with autism), or a pronoun and an auxiliary verb (e.g., person who has aphasia, person who has autism). Some editors, publishers, and institutions require person-first terminology in printed work; others do not. When in doubt, consult the appropriate style manual, read the publisher's submission requirements, or query the potential publisher of your work.

Jargon

Jargon comes from a French word, meaning "gibberish" or "a chattering of birds." In English, the word "jargon" originally meant "confused, unintelligible, incomprehensible language," but gradually acquired a second meaning—"the specialized vocabulary and idioms of people in the same work or profession, such as sportswriters, physicians, computer programmers, and physicists."

Most style manuals and writing authorities distinguish between appropriate and inappropriate jargon. Appropriate jargon is the vocabulary of specialists talking or writing to other specialists. Inappropriate jargon is specialized vocabulary used inappropriately.

Science writing would be impossible without technical vocabulary. Appropriately used technical vocabulary permits writers to communicate complex ideas and concepts in a few words. A writer who uses "diaschisis" does not have to write "effects of an injury remote from the site of injury." A writer who uses "osmosis" does not have to write "passage of fluid through a membrane." If readers know the meaning of such technical words, the writer has communicated efficiently. If readers do not know the term's meaning, the writer has let them down. Appropriate use of technical vocabulary enhances a writer's credibility by suggesting that the writer understands the concepts represented by the terminology and can discuss them in a way that makes sense to others in the specialty.

Now consider the following example, based on a paragraph written by someone who seems to use jargon to impress his readers or to cover his fuzzy thinking. The paragraph appeared in a book intended for readers familiar with medical and neuropsychological lingo, which we do understand. We have changed the wording enough to conceal the identity of the writer, but have preserved, we think, the flavor of what was written:

These elementary actions are instantiated from within abstract structuralized representations presumably maintained in the lexico-motoric interface with the participatory collaboration of two major processes—

a conceptual instantiation module with elementary responsibility for selection of elementary action engrams, and an organizational module with responsibility for the syntactico-temporal characteristics of actions.

The writer of such jargon seems to say, "Look at what a deep thinker I am! See all the high-powered words I know!" Readers seem not to have a place in the writer's purposes. The writer seems bent on impressing readers, not on communicating with them. Such bad jargon —gratuitous use of technical vocabulary—adds to word glut and sabotages clear communication.

Writers of bad jargon use a fancy technical word when a plain word would do because they wish to appear knowledgeable. They do not begin a project, they initialize it, and they do not end it, but finalize it. Their findings do not support a hypothesis, they validate it. They never guess, but often extrapolate. They never report two of anything, but dichotomies of many things. Do not become a member of that club. Do not use a fancy word when a simple one will do.

Be careful about borrowing technical lingo from a specialty unless you are knowledgeable in the specialty. Specialized technical terms have specific meanings, and if you misuse a borrowed technical term, your credibility with knowledgeable readers takes a nosedive. Words such as "synchronize," "extrapolate," "entropy," "catalyst," "continuum," "paradigm," "parameter," and "perimeter" are technical words with precise meanings. Do not use them to replace words such as "match," "surmise," "disorganization," "cause," "range," "measure," and "limits."

If you must use a technical word that may be unknown to many of your readers, define it. Do not define technical words that most readers will know or whose meaning is obvious either from context or because the words are in common use. Most literate adults in the United States know the meaning of words such as "cardiac," "vaccine," and "pulmonary" from medicine, and words such as "neurosis," "obsessive," and "sociopath" from psychology, so you need not define them. If you are unsure about readers' knowledge of a technical word, either define it or substitute a more general word (if the more general word preserves your intended meaning).

Do not shun technical words. But do not pepper your writing with them because you believe that technical words are a path to prestige. Those who know (and that includes knowledgeable readers in your specialty) will see through your scheme and adjust downward their sense of your competence as a writer and scientist. Don't write a fancy word when a simple word will do. Don't write a technical word when an ordinary word will do. Do not borrow highfalutin words from other disciplines simply to impress your readers. The purpose of writing science is to communicate science effectively and efficiently.

Punctuation

Most of us know the basics of punctuation—that periods, question marks, and exclamation points are used to end sentences; that commas are used to mark grammatical boundaries; and that semicolons and colons are used to mark major divisions between grammatical elements. A few of us seem to be less well informed about the specific contexts in which various punctuation marks are appropriate, and many of us are fuzzy on how to punctuate some constructions. Here are some general guidelines for those of us in the latter groups.

End Punctuation

The Period

Put a period at the end of affirmative sentences or mild commands:

> *This is the first in a series of studies.* (Affirmative sentence)

> *Let sleeping dogs lie.* (Mild command)

Put a period after purposeful sentence fragments:

> *This chapter discusses three statistical concepts. The normal distribution. Measures of central tendency. Variability.*

Put a period at the end of indirect questions:

> *I asked Mr. Smith if he had noticed any other symptoms.*

The Question Mark

Put a question mark at the end of direct questions:

> *When did Smith and Jones first publish their findings?*

But not after indirect questions:

> *I wonder when Smith and Jones first published their findings.*

Put a question mark after each of a series of consecutive questions, whether or not they are complete sentences:

What led Smith and Jones to publish their findings? Vanity? Altruism? A desire for tenure?

The Exclamation Point

Put an exclamation point at the end of strong commands or emphatic statements:

Watch where you're going!

That theoretical position is ridiculous!

Exclamation points are (and should be) infrequent in scholarly and scientific writing. When overused, especially in sequences of statements, they lend a frenetic air to your writing and may leave your reader thinking that your sense of urgency is exaggerated.

Do not use (!) to communicate disbelief, sarcasm, or surprise:

Smith and Jones asserted that Hemingway is the 20th century's greatest (!) writer.

Do it with words:

Smith and Jones made the dubious assertion that Hemingway is the 20th century's greatest writer.

The Comma

Commas are the most common of the punctuation marks. They occur in printed materials about twice as often as all other punctuation marks combined. The rules for using commas are more complex than

those for end punctuation, and many writers are unsure of how often to use them and whether to use a comma instead of a semicolon, colon, or dash. The following guidelines may help.

Coordinating Conjunctions

Put a comma before a coordinating conjunction (and, but, or, so, for, nor, yet) that links independent clauses. An independent clause is a grammatical unit that has a subject and a verb and would be a grammatical sentence if capitalized and punctuated correctly:

Mrs. Smith complains of frequent headaches, but her daughter feels that Mrs. Smith is exaggerating their severity.

Do not use a comma when a coordinating conjunction does not link independent clauses, as in the following sentence, which should not have a comma:

Mrs. Smith complains of frequent headaches, and back pain.

Do not use a comma between independent clauses unless they are joined by a coordinating conjunction, as in this sentence, where a comma takes the place of a missing coordinating conjunction. This mistake in punctuation is called a comma splice:

Mrs. Smith complains of frequent headaches, her daughter feels that Mrs. Smith is exaggerating their severity.

A comma is not a strong enough separator in the preceding sentence. There are three alternatives. You might replace the comma with a semicolon:

Mrs. Smith complains of frequent headaches; her daughter feels that Mrs. Smith is exaggerating their severity.

You might separate the clauses into two sentences:

Mrs. Smith complains of frequent headaches. Her daughter feels that Mrs. Smith is exaggerating their severity.

You might add a coordinating conjunction:

Mrs. Smith complains of frequent headaches, but her daughter feels that Mrs. Smith is exaggerating their severity.

When there are commas within independent clauses that are linked by a coordinating conjunction, putting a semicolon before the conjunction may help the reader understand the sentence:

The stimuli were equivalent in length, phonologic complexity, number of syllables, and familiarity; but they were not controlled for imageability, pronouncability, or abstractness.

Better yet, divide such complex sentences into two simpler sentences:

The stimuli were equivalent in length, phonologic complexity, number of syllables, and familiarity. They were not controlled for imageability, pronouncability, or abstractness.

Introductory Material

Put a comma after an introductory element (word, phrase, or clause) that precedes an independent clause:

Though extensive, the literature on sibling rivalry is inconclusive.

When in doubt, apply the more conservative rule.

Furthermore, we cannot assume that these findings can be generalized to the population.

Items in a Series

Put a comma after each of three or more sentence elements in a series, but only if the elements are of equal importance and have the same grammatical form. Commas such as these are called "serial commas" or "Oxford commas":

The results are reliable, unambiguous, and compelling.

The mean scores, mean percentile values, and ranges are given in Table 1.

Some style manuals advise writers not to put a comma before a conjunction that joins the last two items in a series:

The mean scores, mean percentile values and ranges are given in Table 1.

Our advice: Don't leave out this important comma. Readers depend on it.

Coordinate Adjectives

Put a comma between coordinate adjectives—two or more adjectives of equal strength that modify a noun:

A detailed, comprehensive analysis produced different results. (Both "detailed" and "comprehensive" modify "analysis" with equal strength.)

There are two easy ways to decide if two adjectives are coordinate. The first way is to reverse their order. If the new sentence has the same meaning, use a comma:

A comprehensive, detailed analysis produced different results.

The second way is to put "and" between the adjectives. If the resulting sentence reads smoothly, use a comma:

A comprehensive and detailed analysis produced different results.

Do not put commas between noncoordinate adjectives:

Instead of:

Several, detailed analyses failed to change the outcome.

Use:

Several detailed analyses failed to change the outcome. ("Detailed" modifies "analyses"; "several" modifies "detailed analyses.")

Applying the "reversal" and "inserted and" tests yields nonsensical sentences, confirming that commas are not appropriate:

(Reversal) *Detailed several analyses failed to change the outcome.*

(Inserted and) *Several and detailed analyses failed to change the outcome.*

Do not put a comma between a final coordinate adjective and the noun it modi-

fies. This is a common error in manuscripts we have seen submitted for publication. In the following sentence, the comma between "detailed" and "analysis" must go:

A comprehensive, detailed, analysis produced different results.

Essential and Nonessential Sentence Elements

The rule is easy; following it is not. Here is the rule. Use commas to separate nonessential (nonrestrictive) clauses and phrases from the rest of the sentence. Following the rule is complicated because it is often difficult to tell what is essential and what is not in a particular sentence. To find out if a phrase or clause is restrictive, take it out and see what happens to the sentence. If the sentence's core meaning is unchanged, the phrase or clause is nonrestrictive and should be set off by commas:

The data analysis, which was done by technicians in the study center, showed that the experimental group had significantly higher scores than the control group.

Removing "which was done by technicians in the study center" yields:

The data analysis showed that the experimental group had significantly higher scores than the control group.

which has the same core meaning as the original sentence. Now consider the following sentence:

The scores of the participants who received verbal praise were higher than those who received none.

Removing "who received verbal praise" yields:

The scores of the participants were higher than those who received none.

The sentence's core meaning has changed. The clause is essential. It should not be set off with commas.

To Contrast or Limit

Expressions that contrast with or limit previous statements usually are set off by commas:

Mrs. Taylor's reading comprehension is severely impaired, but not her listening comprehension.

The literature is definitive, but only for sophisticated readers.

Quoted Material

Use a comma to separate quoted words from other parts of a sentence:

Einstein said, "God does not play dice with the universe."

The appellation, "a perfect fool," represents the director's competence.

To Clarify Meaning

Sometimes commas are needed to clarify the meaning of a sentence, though no other rule requires them:

Instructors who can, entertain their students as well as inform them.

Without the comma, the sentence is nonsensical:

Instructors who can entertain their students as well as inform them.

Common Errors in Comma Usage

Do not put a comma between the subject and its verb, as in the following sentence:

The participants in the study, were recruited from local middle schools.

Do not put a comma between a verb and its complement, as in the following sentence:

For many years the study of magnetism has been, both neglected and denigrated.

The Semicolon

Semicolons fall between periods and commas in forcefulness. They are weaker than periods, and stronger than commas. They serve several functions.

To Separate Independent Clauses

Semicolons are most often used to separate closely related independent clauses:

The cause of Mrs. Miller's language impairment is not clear; additional testing may be necessary.

Do not use a comma to separate independent clauses in sentences, as in

The cause of Mrs. Miller's language impairment is not clear, additional testing may be necessary.

The comma in the preceding sentence is another example of a comma splice, discussed earlier.

To Separate Independent Clauses Containing Commas, but Joined by a Coordinating Conjunction

Usually sentences with independent clauses linked by a coordinating conjunction require a comma before the conjunction, but when the clauses contain one or more commas, a semicolon placed before the conjunction improves clarity:

When the data were analyzed, the pattern of responses became clearer; but the rate of improvement, although substantial, was not significant.

To Separate Phrases or Clauses with Comma-Containing Elements in a Series

When a sentence contains a series of phrases or clauses that contain commas, use semicolons to separate the series. This helps readers see where each series ends, without having to stop or reread:

The principal investigator recorded, transcribed, and scored participants' responses; coded, tabulated, and organized the data set; and entered the data into a spreadsheet.

To Separate Independent Clauses Linked by Conjunctive Adverbs

Use a semicolon between two independent clauses when the second clause begins with a conjunctive adverb ("however," "nevertheless," "furthermore," "therefore," "con-

sequently," "hence," "likewise," "indeed," "besides," etc.):

After 10 minutes of testing, Mr. Swanson complained that he was extremely tired; therefore, I ended the test and took him back to his room.

Another option is to substitute a period for the semicolon, creating two sentences:

After 10 minutes of testing, Mr. Swanson complained that he was extremely tired. Therefore, I ended the test and took him back to his room.

To Separate Independent Clauses Linked by Transitional Expressions

Use a semicolon between two independent clauses when the second clause begins with a transitional expression ("on the other hand," "as a result," "that is," and the like):

It is clear that Mr. Miller's hearing loss affected his test performance; because of this, these test results are likely to underestimate his true ability.

You can substitute a period for the semicolon:

It is clear that Mr. Miller's hearing loss affected his test performance. Because of this, these test results are likely to underestimate his true ability.

Misuse of Semicolons

Do not use a semicolon between nonindependent clauses or phrases and clauses. Use a comma:

Instead of:

Following instruction; the participants began the experiment.

Use:

Following instruction, the participants began the experiment.

Do not use a semicolon to introduce a list; use a colon:

Each participant met the following selection criteria: English-speaking, more than 50 years old, a native U.S. citizen, literate in English, and living independently.

Note the use of a semicolon in the sentence "Do not use a semicolon to introduce a list; use a colon." If we were to put a coordinating conjunction in the sentence, a comma would be appropriate, as in

Do not use a semicolon to introduce a list, but use a colon.

We could give the assertion more punch by breaking it into two sentences:

Do not use a semicolon to introduce a list. Use a colon.

The Colon

The colon gives stronger separation between adjoining sentence structures than does a semicolon. Colons have several uses.

To Separate Two Independent Clauses

You may use a colon to separate two independent clauses when the first summa-

rizes or explains the second. You may also use a semicolon, a dash, or make two sentences. We prefer any of these alternatives:

The outcome of the study was puzzling: treatment appeared to make participants worse, rather than better.

You can use either uppercase or lowercase for the first letter of the word following the colon. We prefer lowercase. Regardless of which you choose, be consistent throughout your work.

To Introduce a Quotation

Use a colon to introduce a quotation, but only if the material preceding the colon is an independent clause:

Oscar Wilde was not known for his modesty: "I have nothing to declare but my genius."

If the material before the colon is not an independent clause, use a comma:

Kozinski, commenting on failure, said, "If you don't die in the U.S., you underachieve."

To Introduce a Definition

Colons are appropriately used after a phrase or a clause that introduces a definition:

We also counted correct information units: words that were intelligible in context and relevant to the topic.

To Introduce an Appositive

An appositive is a word or a group of words that reiterate an immediately preceding word. An appositive can replace the word it reiterates. You can introduce an appositive with a colon, but only if the material preceding the colon is an independent clause.

The neurosurgeon found it necessary to perform major surgery: an endarterectomy.

To Introduce a List

A colon may introduce a list, but only when the words before the colon constitute an independent clause:

Each participant met the following selection criteria: English-speaking, more than 50 years old, a native U.S. citizen, literate in English, and living independently.

Do not use a colon if the preceding material is not an independent clause:

Instead of:
The stimuli were: circles, squares, rectangles, and trapezoids.

Use:
The stimuli were circles, squares, rectangles, and trapezoids.

It can be tempting to use a colon following words such as "like," "including," "such as," and "consists of," even when the material preceding the colon is not an independent clause. Resist the temptation:

Instead of:
We discovered a number of problems with the transcriptions, including: illegible handwriting, letter omissions, word deletions, and punctuation errors.

Use:
We discovered a number of problems with the transcriptions, including illegible handwriting, letter omissions, word deletions, and punctuation errors.

The Dash

A dash can be used to interrupt a sentence and add information. Use dashes with discretion—overuse lessens their effect and makes text choppy. Dashes and parentheses sometimes serve the same function, but a dash provides a stronger separation:

The participants—those who qualified for the study—were given a form that explained the purposes of the study and the amount of time that would be required from participants.

The participants (those who qualified for the study) were given a form that explained the purposes of the study and the amount of time that would be required from participants.

Parentheses

Use parentheses, like dashes, to interrupt a sentence to add information. Unlike dashes, which emphasize the added information, parentheses tend to de-emphasize what they enclose:

The stimuli (black-and-white line drawings) were divided into two equal sets.

There was a 15-point (nonsignificant) difference between the two groups.

Do not put a comma before an opening parenthesis, even if the sentence element preceding the parenthesis would otherwise require one:

Instead of:

Though the difference was not significant, (p > .05), all but one participant improved from the pretest to the post-test.

Use:

Although the difference was not significant (p > .05), all but one participant improved from the pretest to the post-test.

Comments that fall within a sentence and are enclosed in parentheses are not capitalized and do not end with a closing punctuation mark (period, question mark, exclamation point) even if they form a grammatical sentence:

The difference between the pretest and the post-test (it was not significant) was consistent across all participants.

Free-standing sentences that are within parentheses begin with a capital letter and end with a closing punctuation mark:

The difference was not significant. (However, all but one participant improved from the pretest to the post-test.)

Hyphens

Compound words are combinations of two or more words expressing a single idea (e.g., "pay phone," "rowboat," "lady-in-waiting"). English does not treat compound words consistently. Some are written as separate words ("post office," "cruise ship," "stock market"), some are written as one word ("keyboard," "pineapple," "driveway"), and some are hyphenated ("lady-in-waiting"). Many compounds made up of an adverb and a verb, or a preposition and a noun are written as one word, especially if the combination could cause confusion if written as two words ("underdeveloped," "everlasting," "downstream," "input," "output").

Compound Nouns

Compound nouns are combinations of two nouns. If both nouns in the compound are accented equally ("hound dog," "punch bowl," "book club"), they usually are written as two words. If one member of the compound is less accented ("northwest," "bartender," "suitcase"), the compound usually is written as one word. Dictionaries list common closed (one-word) compound nouns. If you cannot find your compound in the dictionary, write it as two words.

Compound Modifiers

Compound modifiers are another matter. No dictionary could possibly list all the combinations of adjectives, adverbs, and nouns that could create compound modifiers. The U.S. Government Printing Office Style Manual lists 9,000 compound modifiers but does not come close to covering all the possibilities. Knowing how to write compound modifiers can be a hit-or-miss proposition for many writers, but having in hand some general principles and a few rules can make the process less enervating. Hyphens in compound modifiers are used to link the words so that readers cannot misinterpret the compound modifier's intended meaning. Hyphenate them whenever there is any likelihood that an unhyphenated compound will cause your reader to spend time inferring its intended meaning.

Many style manuals are moving away from hyphenation of compound modifiers. They recommend that hyphens be used only when not using them can mislead the reader. A middle ground may be better. When a writer hesitates about hyphenating a modifier, it's likely that the reader also will hesitate unless the construction is hyphenated. So a workable general principle is

"When in doubt, hyphenate."

Some General Principles of Hyphenation

Compound Adjectives. Generally you should hyphenate compound adjectives that precede the noun they modify ("hotter-than-normal weather," "hard-working students"). If the compound is a common one and there is no chance of misinterpretation, you may safely leave the hyphens out (cost of living index, over the counter medications, life insurance policy).

Compound Adverbs and Compounds With "Very." Do not hyphenate compound adverbs that precede the verb they modify ("carefully prepared recipe," "clearly formulated question"), and likewise for compounds beginning with "very" ("very common problem").

Compounds Derived from Adverbs and Verbs or from Prepositions and Nouns. Many of these compounds are written as one word, without hyphens ("overcharged," "everlasting," "underdeveloped," "uphill," "downtrodden"). Those with one-word forms are listed in dictionaries.

Comparatives, Superlatives. Do not hyphenate compounds containing comparatives or superlatives ("better fitting suit," "less common response," "most frequent outcome").

Foreign Phrases. Do not hyphenate compounds consisting of foreign phrases ("ex post facto decision," "post hoc comparisons").

Compound Titles. Do not hyphenate two-word compound titles ("state senator," "vice president," "acting director"). Three-word compound titles usually are hyphenated ("commander-in-chief," "assistant-attorney-general," "chief-executive-officer"). Some three-word compounds may not be hyphenated if the compound is likely to be familiar to the target readership. For example, chief executive officer might not be hyphenated in business publications.

Compounds Containing Letters or Numerals. Fractions expressed in words are hyphenated ("three-fourths," "one-half"), but not words such as "one half" in constructions such as

One half of the group received the treatment and the other half received a placebo.

In this example, "one half" does not represent a fraction, in the mathematical sense of the word.

Hyphenate spelled-out whole numbers from one through ninety-nine (thirty-one, seventy-six), even when they are part of a larger number (one hundred twenty-nine, three thousand, two hundred and sixty-eight).

Hyphenate compounds containing words and numerals when they precede the word they modify (90-minute class, 10-to-1 odds, two-minute drill). Do not hyphenate them if they follow the word they modify ("The class lasted for 90 minutes," "The odds were 10 to 1.")

If the numeric word in a compound modifier is possessive, do not hyphenate the compound (two weeks' work, 40 hours' pay).

Hyphenate combinations of letters and numerals that identify brands, models, or types of manufactured goods (DC-10, 4-by-4, MP-III).

Suspended Hyphens

When two or more compound modifiers in sequence have a common referent, some writers omit the referent in all but the last modifier (e.g., four- and five-year curricula, 30- 60- or 90-minute periods, inter- and intra-examiner reliability). But be careful. Suspended hyphens make comprehension more difficult for readers. They leave readers in limbo about the referent until they reach the completed compound at the end of the sequence. Then they must mentally backtrack to fill in the gaps left by the suspended hyphens. This is especially likely for sequences of more than two or three compound modifiers. The writer eliminates two or three redundant words, but the reader spends far more time in dealing with the discontinuities created than they would spend in reading the missing words. Many editors dislike suspended hyphens, so our advice is, "don't use them, they're not worth it."

Instead of *four- and five-year curricula,* write *four-year and five-year curricula.*

Instead of *30- 60- or 90-minute periods,* write *30-minute, 60-minute, or 90-minute periods.*

Do not separate prefixes and stems of nonhyphenated compound words and then use suspended hyphens (under- and overpass access, in- and outpatient treatment) in sequences of such words.

What To Do If You Are Not Sure of Hyphenation

If a compound could have a meaning different from the one you intend, hyphenate. Ask yourself if the compound you intend to use could have another meaning. For example, an "old-house painter" paints old houses, but an "old house painter" is an old person who paints houses. A "new car dealer" is a car dealer who is new to the city, but a "new-car dealer" is one who sells new cars. A "large-animal clinic" is a clinic that specializes in large animals. A "large animal clinic" is an animal clinic that is large. Always hyphenate if not hyphenating could generate confusion.

References

Bresnan, J., Dingare, S., & Manning, C. (2001). *Soft constraints mirror hard constraints: Voice and person in English and Lummi. Proceedings of the LFG '01 Conference.* Stanford, CA: CSLI Publications.

Fowler, H., & Fowler, F. (1908). *The King's English.* London, UK: Clarendon Press.

Morrision, B. (2005, August 5). Black day for the blue pencil. *The Guardian.* Retrieved from http://www.theguardian.com/books/2005/aug/06/featuresreviews.guardian review1

Quirk, R., Greenbaum, S., Leech, G., & Svartvik, J. (1985). *A comprehensive grammar of the English language.* Harlow, Essex, UK: Longman.

Xiao, R., McEnery, T., & Qian, Y. (2006). Passive constructions in English and Chinese: A corpus-based contrastive study. *Languages in Contrast, 6,* 9–49.

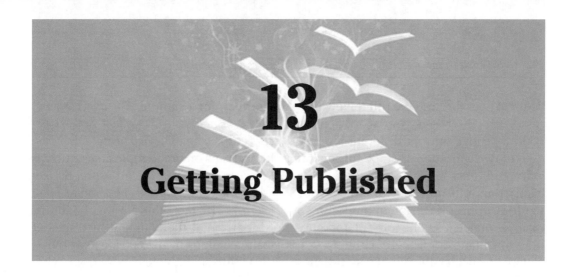

13

Getting Published

*"Peer review . . . is the process through which journal articles are reviewed,
revised and published in the pursuit of disseminating new knowledge."*

—Eimear Muir-Cochrane

The Changing Face of Publication

The Internet has disrupted scientific publishing as it has all other media, and the process of publishing and accessing research reports is changing rapidly. The scope of these changes can be glimpsed in the special issue of the preeminent journal *Nature* on the future of publishing (*Nature*, 2013, vol. 495). The ability to share information globally with little cost has led to the development of alternate forms of publication that have become central to the scientific enterprise. The National Institutes of Health (NIH) now require all grantees to make their peer-reviewed publications available to the public free of charge through the PubMed Central online archive. The full texts of 11% of articles published in 2011 were available immediately online in Open Access journals (OA) (Laakso & Björk, 2012).

Not everything has changed, however. Note the reference to peer review in the NIH requirement to make a report available. Peer review remains an impor-

tant part of the publishing process, and so we will discuss it later in this chapter. You will need to interact with editors to have your work published in most journals, and this process is discussed as well. The first step is to choose where to submit your masterpiece.

Issues to Consider When Choosing a Journal

Align With Journal's Mission and Scope

Every peer-reviewed journal has a journal website that describes the journal's mission and scope. Be sure to read these prior to submitting your manuscript for review. If you are unsure if your manuscript is a good fit with the journal, then e-mail the editor and ask. Include a copy of your abstract to give the editor a brief overview of your work. Editors welcome these types of inquiries; it saves them and you precious time. It is much better to find out that your manuscript is not suitable before it goes through the full review process. If an editor says your work is not a good fit, move on to a different journal. You may send the abstract to several journals at once to save time. If you hear back from multiple editors that your work is appropriate for submission to their journal, chose one journal and submit your manuscript there. How do you choose? Consider the journal's audience and reputation.

Consider Your Audience

When considering the audience, think about the professionals who read the journal. The American Speech-Language-Hearing Association (ASHA) publishes four journals: *Journal of Speech, Language, and Hearing Research* (JSLHR), *American Journal of Speech-Language Pathology* (AJSLP), *American Journal of Audiology* (AJA), and *Language, Speech, and Hearing Services in Schools* (LSHSS). Each of these journals has a different scope and mission. JSLHR publishes research studies related to speech, language, and hearing, and of the four journals it has the broadest scope. AJSLP and AJA publish research that is more clinically focused than that in JSLHR. LSHSS publishes work of interest to those working in the schools. ASHA members can access these journals online free of charge as a member benefit, and therefore these journals represent the most likely places for speech-language pathologists (SLPs) and audiologists to read your work. ASHA also issues *Perspectives* publications associated with each special interest group (SIG); these publications are available to members of any SIG. There are, of course, many other journals out there that are not published by ASHA that might be appropriate for your work. Some of these journals focus on specific disorders, for example, *Ear and Hearing*, the *Journal of Fluency Disorders*, or the *Journal of Autism and Developmental Disorders*. Others focus on broad topic areas, such as *Neurology*, *Journal of the Acoustical Society of America*, or the *Journal of Communication Disorders*. In fact, the National Library of Medicine at the National Institutes of Health catalogs over 5,600 journals (NIH, 2014). With so many to choose from, what additional factors should authors consider, aside from mission, scope, and audience?

Journal Reputation

"The only happy author in this world is he who is below the care of reputation."
(Washington Irving)

Should you be in the happy state of having several journals vying to publish you work, you might consider the reputation or ranking of the journals to determine which to choose. In addition to the opinions of colleagues and mentors, computer algorithms can give insight into the quality of work published in a journal. Impact Factor, introduced by Institute for Scientific Information (now Thomson-Reuters) in 1975, is the ratio of the number of citations made to articles published in the journal during the previous 2 years divided by the number of citable articles. An impact factor of 3 for 2011 means on average each article published in the journal during 2009–2010 was cited three times in 2011. Impact factors for many journals can be found on the Web of Science. Variations include 5-year impact factors and elimination of self-references. Impact factors can give insight into the importance that the journal has on a given research field but can be distorted by several factors. Thomson-Reuters notes that "the impact factor should not be used without careful attention to the many phenomena that influence citation rates."

Eigenfactor is a more complex method of ranking journals developed by Bergstrom and colleagues (2008) that attempts to take into account the ranking of the journals from which the citations originate. Eigenfactor.org lists values for many journals. SCImago Journal Rank (SJR indicator) is another measure of scientific influence, and listings can be found at http://www.scimagojr.com/

The Submission and Review Process

Submitting Your Manuscript

After deciding where to submit your work, you have to decide what type of article you are submitting. The options vary by journal and are described on the journal webpage. Some of the more common types of articles are Research, Clinical Focus, Brief Reports, and Research Notes. Research manuscripts report the results of experiments or investigations that may or may not have clinical utility. Clinical Focus articles address aspects of clinical interventions; these articles may also address protocols for clinical measurement. Brief Reports are, as the title suggests, shorter than a typical research article and may be used to report data that are of particular interest to the journal's audience, but for which there are not as yet enough data to warrant a full research article. Research Notes typically address potential improvements in research methodology or new methods. If you are not sure what type of article your manuscript is, write the editor and ask.

The next step is to review the journal's guidelines for authors. These guidelines are available on the journal website, and they stipulate the format that needs to be followed for manuscripts submitted to the journal. For example, author guidelines will define the format for citations, specify the placement of figures and tables, and tell you if the document should be single or double spaced. Pay close attention to these seemingly minor details; failure to follow the author guidelines can mean an "instant reject" of your manuscript without review.

Most journals require electronic submission of manuscripts, via online software platforms designed for this purpose. Access to the online submission platform is available on the journal's website. Submitting your manuscript involves uploading a series of files and completing online forms. It is wise to review the list of files required and the information requested before actually submitting your manuscript, because some platforms require separate files for the title page, abstract, manuscript, tables, and figures. If the journal conducts blind reviews, the journal will ask you to submit a "blind copy" of your documents that does not contain any author information.

The submission software will prompt you to enter your manuscript title, author names and affiliations, and manuscript type. You will be required to enter a list of key words that will be used to index your article once it is published (more on key words in the Helping Search Engines Find Your Work section below and Chapter 8, The Title). You will be prompted to answer a series of questions about research ethics and your study. You will be asked to verify that you have Institutional Review Board (IRB) approval; that all authors contributed to the final document; that there are no conflicts of interest; and that you have not submitted the work elsewhere. You will also be asked if the research was funded and if so by what organization. If you are not prompted for this information, then you should include it in a cover letter to the editor. Authors have the option of submitting a cover letter to the editor, and you should always do so. These brief letters are a professional courtesy to the editor, introducing your manuscript and thanking them for coordinating the review process. If there are potential peer reviewers who you think would be particularly biased against your work, you should name these people in the cover letter and request that they not review your work. This decision is at the editor's discretion, but most will honor these requests.

Occasionally, you may want to include in your manuscript figures or charts that have been published elsewhere by other researchers. In order to include such work in your manuscript, you must ask for copyright permission to do so. This involves contacting the publisher of the work you wish to include and requesting permission to use the work. Copyright permission can be requested from many publishers via the website http://www.copyright.com, otherwise contact the publisher directly using e-mail or phone information from their website. Some copyright permissions are granted free of charge, whereas others cost money. Be sure to ask about the price.

Some journals allow submission of supplementary material such as videos, datasets, and audio recordings. The use of supplementary material is growing with the increase in online access to journals, but it is best to consult with your editor on the wisdom and pitfalls of supplementary materials.

Once you have entered all the required information, answered all the questions, and uploaded your document files, the software will generate a pdf document for your review. Once you hit the submit button, you cannot change the manuscript, so review the document carefully. You should save a copy of this document on your computer prior to submitting it. Once you submit, the software generates a manuscript reference number; refer to this number in any subsequent interactions with the editor or staff at the journal. You should also receive a confirmation e-mail stating that your manuscript was submitted.

Once the manuscript is submitted, journal administrators review it for compliance with the guidelines for authors. Once your manuscript passes this initial vetting process, it goes to the editor.

Behind the Scenes: What Happens to Your Manuscript After It Is Submitted

Editors review all submissions and decide to either (a) immediately reject the manuscript or (b) assign an associate editor (AE) to the submission, based on topic expertise. The most common reasons for an immediate rejection are that (a) the manuscript is not a good fit for the journal, or (b) the writing is so bad that the manuscript is incomprehensible as written.

What It Means to Be "Peer Reviewed"

The peer review process is the foundation upon which the house of science is built. Peer review is a vetting process in which scholars evaluate the work of other scholars, to ensure that the questions asked are interesting and useful; that the author has accurately placed his or her work within the context of what is already known; that the methodology is sound; and that the results add to what we know about the topic. Peer review is a quality control process that helps authors and editors work together to maintain the quality of the scientific literature.

The AE coordinates the peer review process. The AE assigns peer reviewers who read the manuscript and comment on it. These reviewers are researchers in the field with expertise on the manuscript topic. The reviewers typically have 1 month to submit their review. The AE then summarizes the reviews and adds comments. The AE's summary and all peer reviews are forwarded to the editor, who evaluates the manuscript based on the reviews and his or her own expertise. The editor makes the final decision regarding the manuscript and responds to the author with comments, the AE summary, and the peer reviews. Editors can accept the manuscript, reject the manuscript, or ask the author to revise and resubmit the manuscript.

If the editor decides to accept your manuscript, you may be asked for some minor changes to the document prior to sending it on to be proofed by the journal staff. These minor changes typically involve adding or deleting figures and tables and rewording of the text. Acceptance after the first round of peer review is quite rare, and means that only minor changes are necessary prior to publication.

More often, the editor will ask you to revise and resubmit your manuscript. A revise and resubmit decision means that the journal is still interested in publishing your work, provided that you address issues and concerns noted by the peer reviewers, AE, and editor. You will receive an e-mail from the editor containing written comments from the editor, AE, and

all reviewers. Be sure to address all of the comments, even if you believe some are mistaken. You may choose not to follow through with particular suggestions from the reviewers, but you must explain why you did not do so. Do not simply ignore the suggestions; good editors will go back and make sure you have addressed the reviewers' suggestions by making changes or explaining why changes are not appropriate.

Copying the editor's e-mail response into a word processing document allows you to address all the comments in an organized manner. For each suggestion, write an author response directly beneath it. Continue until all the suggestions have been addressed. Be sure to include these responses in your letter to the editor that accompanies your resubmission. Editors and AEs will appreciate your attention to detail. You are having a written interaction with the editor, AE, and reviewers, so respond professionally. Make it a priority to respond promptly.

At this point, the AE may send the revised manuscript out for another round of peer review, or the AE may review the revised manuscript. This is at the AE's discretion. If the first round of reviews suggested major revisions, then the AE will likely elect to send the revised manuscript out for review again. AEs can be influenced by the authors' thoroughness in responding to feedback; it is in the authors' best interest to be as thorough as possible in addressing the reviews. Making a clear case may allow the AE to judge the manuscript without having to send it out for another round of review.

Editors can also decide to reject your manuscript. The most frequent reason for rejection is that the manuscript does not fit with the scope or mission of the journal. Your best recourse is to find another journal to publish your work. Use the feedback you received from the editor and reviewers to strengthen your manuscript prior to submitting it to another journal. Another reason for rejection is the presence of a "fatal flaw" in the manuscript, usually in the methodology. If this is the reason for rejection, then do not send the flawed manuscript to another journal. It will get rejected there, too. Instead, use the comments to rework your study and improve it prior to submitting it elsewhere.

The Final Stretch: Preparing the Manuscript for Publication

Once your manuscript is accepted, it then goes through another vetting process by journal administrators. Administrators check to make sure all the files are uploaded and in the correct order. They then pass the manuscript to the production staff for editing. The production staff produces page proofs with queries to the author embedded in them. For example, the production staff will check citations, and if they cannot find one as you submitted it, they will ask you to correct it. Be sure to address each query, and respond promptly. You will then be asked to approve the page proofs. You can make punctuation and other minor corrections but the time for editing is past. The production staff completes the final edits, and your manuscript is published. Journal websites often have a section called "online first" or "newly published articles" where they place articles that they have accepted for publication. This may be the first place to see your study in print; the "official" copy with volume numbers and page numbers may come a few days or weeks later.

Helping Search Engines Find and Index Your Work

Gone are the days when graduate students spent hours in the stacks of the library, reading through hard copies of journals, looking for citations to bolster the arguments in their manuscripts. These days, almost all research articles are available online, which has important implications for authors. You want to write your title, abstract, and key word lists to maximize the likelihood that your work will appear in online searches, so that people will find your work, download it, and read it. This process is called *academic search engine optimization* (ASEO).

It is important to have a general understanding of how search engines such as Google Scholar and PubMed "find" articles and rank them in their search results. Both of these search engines use mathematical algorithms that rank articles by weighting particular characteristics of the article. For example, Google Scholar uses an article's relevance to the search query, number of citations, author names, and title to determine how articles are ranked in search results (Beel, Gipp, & Wilde, 2010). Other search engines use different characteristics to determine article rankings. Of all these characteristics, relevance is the most important and the most commonly used.

Relevance is determined by the presence of words that match the search query in the article title, abstract, key word list, and text. This is why you should choose your key words carefully. Once chosen, make sure these key words appear in your article's title, abstract, and text. If asked to provide a brief author biography, put the key words in there as well. Some search engines provide specific vocabulary lists that they use to search topics and rank results; using these terms can increase your article's relevance and rankings in search results. The ERIC database has lists of descriptors that allow for more specific searching of a topic. For example, for the topic of "reading," there are 48 descriptors, including "dyslexia," "story telling," and "reading fluency." If your article is about dyslexia, then using "dyslexia" rather than "reading" as a key word will likely improve the relevance of your article in searches for "dyslexia." The PubMed search engine uses Medical Subject Headings (MeSH) to categorize research topics. MeSH terms are arranged in hierarchical "trees" from general to specific terms. Here again, using a MeSH term will increase your article's relevance rating, because these are the terms that PubMed uses to rank articles.

Publication Ethics

There are rules that all authors should be aware of:

- The work you submit is your own.
- Co-authors have made contributions to the work (see the Publication Manual of the APA for specific guidelines for authorship).
- Cite your sources, give credit to the work of others, and do not plagiarize.
- Document your Institutional Review Board (IRB) approval for human subjects research.
- Acknowledge any financial support for your work.
- Acknowledge any possible conflicts of interest, either financial or personal.
- Submit to only one journal at a time.

- Once your work is published, do not submit the identical work to another journal.
- Editors and peer reviewers are typically not paid and do this work as a service to the profession, so treat them with respect.

Final Thoughts

Reading and reviewing the work of others can improve your own work. Being a good peer reviewer takes time and practice. It can be challenging to write constructive reviews that help authors make their work better. Being a peer reviewer trains you to look at manuscripts with a critical eye, and can make your own work better. Consider volunteering to be a peer reviewer by making your desire known to the journal editor in a brief e-mail that indicates your areas of expertise.

Finally, the review process is not personal. Try not to take the reviewer's comments personally. Their comments address the manuscript, not you as a person.

References

Beel, J., Gipp, B., & Wilde, E. (2010). Academic search engine optimization (ASEO): Optimizing scholarly literature for Google Scholar & Co. *Journal of Scholarly Publishing, 41,* 176–190.

Bergstrom, C. T., West, J. D., & Wiseman, M. A. (2008). The Eigenfactor™ Metrics. *Journal of Neuroscience, 28*(45), 11433–11434.

Laakso, M., & Björk, B-C. (2012). Anatomy of open access publishing: A study of longitudinal development and internal structure. *BMC Medicine, 10,* 124.

Muir-Cochrane, E. (2013). What do journal editors want? . . . and everything you wanted to know about the peer review process for journal publication. *Nursing and Health Sciences, 15,* 263–264.

National Institutes of Health. Retrieved from http://www.nlm.nih.gov/bsd/num_titles .html

Nature.com. (2013). A new page: A special issue of *Nature* looks at the transformation taking place in scientific publishing. *Nature, 495,* 409–544.

Thomson-Reuters. (1994). *The Thomson-Reuters Impact Factor.* Retrieved from http://wok info.com/essays/impact-factor/

14
The Writing Process

"Inspiration is for amateurs; the rest of us just show up and get to work."

—Chuck Close (Fig, 2009)

The purpose of this chapter is to provide some resources to assist you in the writing process. We've organized it into four sections. The first section describes resources to help get started and keep going with the writing process. The second section contains suggestions for making the writing process as efficient as possible. The third section describes resources for those who incorporate writing into their classes and for students who take writing classes. In the conclusion, we provide some guidelines that have helped us with our writing and we hope will help you with yours.

Resources for Getting Started and Keeping Going

It can be difficult to begin a writing project, particularly if you have been away from writing for awhile. There is no "trick" to getting started again—just put words on the page. When your thesis advisor or professor says, "I don't care how lousy the draft is, just get me something on paper and I will comment on it," they are giving you a kick-start on the road to writing. Anne Lamott calls it a "shitty first draft, . . . the child's draft, where you let it all pour out and then let it romp all over the place . . . knowing that you can shape it later" (Lamott, 1994, p. 22). The most basic step in getting started is to put something—anything—on paper. One word, then a sentence, then some more sentences. For the first draft, shove your internal editor out the door and just write. You can't edit or change something until it is on the page or screen in front of you.

What if you have some serious writer's block, and you psych yourself out about writing even before you can get started? You start thinking of all the writing that you need to ever do in your career instead of the paper in front of you. A big part of getting started is not sabotaging yourself before you begin. Writing can be a lonely process, and an especially difficult one to start if you have writer's block. So, what do you do? Get yourself some writing friends, as Paul Silvia (2007) suggests. Find one or two colleagues with an interest in writing, and form a writing group. Meet biweekly to set individual writing goals and shared progress toward those goals. The point is that this type of group keeps you accountable to meeting your goals. If you form a writing group, it must be with people you trust.

If you don't feel comfortable forming a group with your work colleagues or fellow students, consider joining one of many online writing clubs. There are many such clubs; some are focused academic writing (e.g., Academic Ladder, Academic Muse), whereas others address fiction, poetry, and other types of creative writing (e.g., Scribophile, TheNextBigWriter, WritersCafe). You can remain anonymous in these clubs by writing under a pen name. The functions and operating principles of the groups vary. Common functions include providing accountability, social support, a sense of community, constructive feedback on writing, and writing advice.

Although there is no "one right way" to approach writing, one common piece of advice is to avoid binge writing. Binge writing is the opposite of writing a little every day. If you put off writing until you need to work overtime to meet a deadline, chances are the writing process will be onerous, fraught with anxiety. It is natural to avoid onerous activities, particularly those that make us anxious or fearful of failure. Binge writing creates a vicious cycle: I do not write until external or internal pressures force me to binge to get it done, but after binging I am sick of writing so I avoid it, and the cycle repeats. Better to write a bit every day—20 minutes or so—and come back to it in a positive mood the next day. As you finish a writing session, you can maintain your momentum by writing two to three ideas to start with next time. These ideas will help you get started when you begin your next writing session; you will not waste valuable time trying to remember what you were going to write next.

Suggestions for Making the Writing Process More Efficient

Nothing derails writing like being interrupted by others. Figure out what time of day works best for you to write undisturbed, and then schedule yourself to write at that time of day. Put writing on your schedule and guard it like a treasure. No, you can't meet at that time because it is during your writing time. Treat writing time like class time—no one would suggest that you skip class to attend a meeting. When you start thinking of writing time as flexible time, it often gets flexed right out of the schedule.

Steven King notes that, "The closed door is your way of telling the world and yourself that you mean business; you have made a serious commitment to write and intend to walk the walk as well as talk the talk" (King, 2000, p. 155). We asked a few colleagues from different universities where and when they write. Notice how some of their suggestions echo that of King:

- "I write at night, after the kids are in bed."
- "At work, with the door closed."
- "In the morning, before anyone else is up."
- "If I have to get some writing done at work, I close the door and turn my office light off, so people think I am not there."
- "I've found that putting a 'do not disturb' sign on my office door does not dissuade people from interrupting me. So, if I really have to write, I put a sign up on my door that says, 'on conference call until _____.' This works!"

- "I try to write at the same time every day."
- "I write at the coffee shop. I like the background noise and anonymity." (But be sure to buy a cup every hour or so!)

Some colleagues write in the morning, at home, before heading in to work. This ensures that they are not interrupted when they write. Writing in the morning gives a sense of accomplishment early in the day, and this in turn motivates them to continue writing the next day. The important thing is to reflect on your opportunities and commitments, find times where you can write undisturbed, and get writing into your schedule.

Citation managers also help improve writing efficiency. Citation managers are software programs that organize your citations, create searchable indexes of your citations, and format your citation lists for manuscripts. Citation management software can format your in-text and citation lists in many different formats (e.g., APA, MLA) with relative ease; this ability is useful if you have written your manuscript in APA format but elect to submit it to a journal that uses MLA format. Even though citation managers take a bit of time to learn how to use, this time is well spent. One caution: as with any software, citation managers are not infallible. They are not error free. Always check the citation list generated for accuracy in form and content. There are many citation managers available; some cost money (e.g., EndNote, RefWorks), whereas others are free (e.g., Zotero, Citavi). Regardless of which citation manager you use, the more you use it, the more useful it will become, as you build a library of citations. Many universities provide citation managers to students and faculty free of charge; your

university librarian will know which one your university uses.

If you do not have access to a citation manager, the best way to create your citation list and to ensure that your in-text citations are done correctly is to consult the style manual that the journal uses. Although many style manuals exist, the two that are encountered most frequently in Communication Sciences and Disorders (CSD) journals are the manuals of the American Psychological Association (APA) and the Modern Language Association (MLA). The ASHA journals discussed in the previous chapter follow the rules of APA style. When creating a citation list, seemingly minor issues (e.g., should I order the citations alphabetically or by when they occur in the text?) are exactly what writers need to pay attention to. Not following style rules can lead to an immediate rejection of your manuscript, so it's worth getting it right. Every university library will have multiple copies of the APA and MLA style manuals; make use of them. Finally, many online resources exist to guide new writers in the details of APA style; our favorite is Douglas Degelman's (2013) six-page concise summary of APA style.

Writing Resources for Teachers and Students

I teach a *Writing in the Disciplines* course at my university. One of the main purposes of the course is to mentor students through the writing process. Students write on a clinical topic in CSD. They produce initial drafts, they peer review and edit each other's work, and then they write a final draft. We also do a lot of writing beyond formal research papers. I use

1-minute papers (Angelo & Cross, 1993) to assess student knowledge and gauge the level of engagement with course material. One-minute papers involve posing a question or issue to the class, and having students write a response in 1 minute. I review their responses prior to the next class and adjust the lesson plan to address any misconceptions or inaccuracies that were present in the papers. Students also produce written products when they do group work; these group reports allow me to assess their knowledge and how well their group is working together.

John Bean's (2011) book, *Engaging Ideas*, provides teachers with excellent methods of providing feedback to students about writing without getting bogged down with the grading. Purdue's Online Writing Lab (Purdue OWL, 2015) contains a variety of resources for writing teachers and writers, including exercises related to the writing process. The Writing Matters newsletters (University of Hawai'i at Manoa, 2015) contain information on designing assignments, responding to written work, creating peer review forms, and many other topics useful for writing teachers.

Sometimes it's helpful to read a well-written article or two before writing your own paper. Articles that have won ASHA editor's awards are good examples. Lists of these articles are published in the ASHA *Leader*; keep the lists in your class notes, and refer students to these articles as needed.

There are many books available on the writing process itself. We took an informal poll of colleagues, and two books seemed to make everyone's list of "good books about writing." These books were Robert Boice's (1990) *Professors As Writers: A Self-Help Guide to Productive Writing*, and Wendy Belcher's (2009) *Writing Your Journal Article in Twelve Weeks: A Guide to Academic Publishing Success*. I would add Paul Silvia's (2007) *How to Write a Lot* to this list of books that address the writing process in detail.

Guidelines for the Writing Process

- Be confident that you can write and get it done. Do not psych yourself out before you start, just get to work.
- Figure out what time of day works best for you to write undisturbed.
- Find a trustworthy writing buddy to keep you on track and accountable.
- You can improve your writing by reading about the writing process.
- Be comfortable with "shitty first drafts," knowing that there are many better drafts to come.
- Guard your writing time. Put "writing" on your weekly schedule and stick to it.
- Ban binge writing.
- Write a little every day.

References

Angelo, T., & Cross, K. P. (1993). *Classroom assessment techniques: A handbook for college teachers* (2nd ed.). San Francisco, CA: Jossey-Bass.

Bean, J. (2011). *Engaging ideas: The professor's guide to integrating writing, critical thinking, and active learning in the classroom* (2nd ed.). San Francisco, CA: Jossey-Bass.

Belcher, W. L. (2009). *Writing your journal article in twelve weeks: A guide to academic publishing success*. Thousand Oaks, CA: Sage.

Boice, R. (1990). *Professors as writers: A self-help guide to productive writing*. Stillwater, OK: New Forums Press.

Degelman, D. (2013). *APA style essentials*. Retrieved from http://www.vanguard.edu/psychology/wp-content/uploads/2013/02/apastyleessentials.pdf

Fig, J. (2009). *Inside the painter's studio* (p. 42). New York, NY: Princeton Architectural Press.

King, S. (2001). *On writing*. New York, NY: Scribner.

Lamott, A. (1994). *Bird by bird: Some instructions on writing and life*. New York, NY: Pantheon Books.

Purdue Online Writing Lab. (2015). Retrieved from https://owl.english.purdue.edu/owl/

Silvia, P. (2007). *How to write a lot: A practical guide to productive academic writing*. Washington, DC: American Psychological Association.

University of Hawaii at Manoa. (2015). Retrieved from http://manoa.hawaii.edu/mwp/mwp-office/about-us/program-research/writing-matters

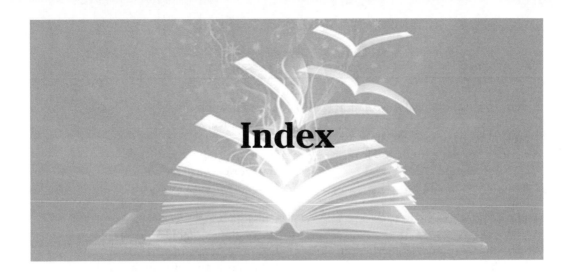

Index

Note: Page numbers in **bold** reference non-text material.

α (alpha), 29–30, 39
χ^2 (chi-square), **27**
η (eta, partial eta), 29–30
1–minute paper, 202

A

Abbreviations
  in abstract, 116–117
  in graphs, 85
  in tables, 37, **37**, 42, 44, **44**, 45, 55–56
  in titles, 105–106, 107
  of compound title, 189
Abstract
  abbreviations in, 116–117
  active voice, 119
  clutter in, 117–118, 120
  indicative, 114
  informative, 114–115
  length, 120
  numbers in, 117
  opening, 117–119
  style of, 115–120
  symbols in, 116–117
  tables in, 119
  units in, 116
  verb tense, 119–120
Academic search engine optimization,
    196–197
Accepted manuscript, 196
Acronyms. *See* Abbreviations
Active voice,
  in abstract, 119
  in method section, 17, 23

tutorial on, 161–165
  See also Passive voice
"Additional research needed," in
    discussion, 91–92
Adjective
  clutter, 158–159
  empty, 160
  hedging, 94
  nominalized, 155–156
  referent for pronoun, 170
  repeated, 159–160, 160n1
  smothered, 158–159
Adjectives, comma between coordinate,
    182–183
Adverb
  clutter, 157–158
  smothered, 157–158
  split compound verb, 173–174
  split infinitive, 172
AJA (*American Journal of Audiology*), 192
AJSLP (*American Journal of Speech-Language
    Pathology*), 192
Alignment, table, 45–48, **47**, **48**
Allied health disciplines, writing in, 2
"Almost," as limiting modifier, 167
Alpha value (α), 29–30, 39
Ambiguous modifier, 167–168
American Journal of Audiology (AJA), 192
*American Journal of Speech-Language
    Pathology* (AJSLP), 192
American Psychological Association (APA)
  authorship requirements, 197
  statistical test report format, 31
  style manual, 201